Transforming Healthcare

Harnessing the Power of Artificial Intelligence for Enhanced Patient Care

SB Wade

Table of Contents

Introduction

Imagine lying on a hospital bed, scared and uncertain. Your symptoms are puzzling, your medical history is complicated, and you have a sinking feeling that the doctors are shooting in the dark. Then, an Artificial Intelligence (AI) program, having read through millions of case studies and having been updated on the latest medical research, suggests a precise, targeted treatment for you. You follow it, and your symptoms begin to recede within days. Almost too good to be true, yet, as of 2023, an AI chatbot has already assisted doctors in treating over 3 million people. Welcome to the future of healthcare (Jennings, 2023).

You've come here out of concern, feeling frustrated with the current state of healthcare or a provider drowning in paperwork and outdated protocols. Whether you're a patient who's tired of the bureaucratic, impersonal, and error-prone healthcare system or a healthcare provider drowning in paperwork and outdated protocols, you know something must change. The current healthcare system is fraught with inefficiency, misdiagnoses, and even medical errors that put real people's lives at risk. It's the provenance of collective anxiety, an open wound in modern society, begging desperately for a real solution.

This book serves as a guide to the new reality. Within its pages, you'll discover

- **Simplifications of Technical Jargon:** Understand complex concepts like Machine Learning (ML), Natural Language Processing (NLP), and system and information-based interoperability without needing a Ph.D. in computer science.

- **Patient Benefits:** Learn how AI could make your next visit to the doctor quicker, more accurate, and far less stressful.

- **Solving Common Complaints:** We'll tackle the issues patients complain about most often—the high cost of healthcare, long waiting times, access to care, impersonal care, and the maze of insurance—and demonstrate how AI offers tangible solutions.

- **Challenges and Risks:** AI isn't a magic bullet. We need to understand the limitations and ethical considerations of which we need to be aware.

- **Quality Control:** Learn how AI systems are trained and the regulatory safeguards put in place to ensure they act in your best interest.

- **Testimonials:** Hear compelling stories, including celebrity experiences, where AI in healthcare made a life-changing or life-saving difference.

By the time you turn the last page, you'll have a comprehensive understanding of how AI could revolutionize healthcare, making it more efficient, patient-friendly, and, ultimately, more effective at caring for you. You'll also gain a realistic view of the challenges and ethical complexities that come with integrating machine intelligence into a sector as sensitive as healthcare.

Why should you trust this book? We've seen the pitfalls and promises firsthand, and we're here to share that hard-won knowledge with you. This isn't speculative fiction; it's a roadmap to an already unfolding future.

Before artificial intelligence information was synthesized and made accessible, patients and healthcare providers had to wade through fragmented data, academic papers, and speculation. It was very difficult to imagine all the possibilities. But now, all the information is at your fingertips, presented in an accessible format.

This is not just another book; this is your companion guide to the future of healthcare, a future that is already here. Are you ready to be a part of it?

Chapter 1:

The Current Landscape of Technology in Healthcare

This chapter will take you on a journey through the evolving landscape of healthcare technology. From the role that rudimentary technology has played to the explosive emergence of Artificial Intelligence, we will examine the transformative power of technology in the healthcare industry. Through real-life case studies, we'll understand the scope and limitations of the current systems and shed light on the promise that AI holds to revolutionize healthcare as we know it.

The Life-Saving Potential of Digital Resources

In 2017, Vipin Khadse found himself in a precarious situation. A medical student at a university in India, on his way to becoming a qualified doctor—he was on the train when a woman went into labor. The situation turned out to be very complicated; the baby was in a breech position, a potentially fatal complication if not managed correctly. With no other medical professionals around and limited resources, Khadse did what might have seemed unthinkable years ago—he turned to an instant messaging app (Whatsapp) for medical consultation. Following remote guidance from senior doctors, he successfully delivered the baby, turning what could have been a tragic event into a miraculous one. Technology became an invaluable resource, an extension of medical knowledge and expertise, and it probably saved two lives that day.

Switch continents and move forward a few years to a hospital room in Tokyo where a 60-year-old woman lay with what doctors believed was acute myeloid leukemia. The treatments they had administered were doing nothing to improve her condition, leaving them stumped and desperate. As a last-ditch effort, the team plugged her medical records into IBM's Watson, a medically trained AI capable of reading and analyzing over 20 million cancer research papers in less than 10 minutes. Watson analyzed her data and concluded that she had a rare form of leukemia that had been overlooked. A revised treatment plan, recommended by Watson and vetted by the doctors, was promptly initiated, which led to her improvement. Here again, technology—in the form of sophisticated artificial intelligence—stepped in to change the course of a patient's life.

So, what do these two stories teach us about the state of technology in healthcare? In the first instance, even a simple messaging app, often taken for granted in our daily lives, became a crucial lifeline in a medical emergency. In the second, a far more complex technology—AI—was able to sift through many mountains of data to provide a diagnosis that human doctors had missed. These are not isolated incidents but rather indicators of a seismic shift in healthcare.

The question that naturally arises is: If this is what is possible now, what does the future hold? As we dig deeper into this chapter, we'll examine the various ways technology has been enhancing healthcare and how the rise of AI presents unprecedented possibilities—and challenges.

Bridging The Gap: From Traditional Tech to AI

These two gripping stories epitomize the dual narrative of healthcare technology today. In the first, we see a relatively rudimentary but incredibly useful form of technology—an instant messaging app—enabling remote consultations in emergency scenarios. In the second, we delve into the advanced capabilities of AI, a technology that promises to reshape the very foundations of healthcare, capable of complex diagnostics and personalized treatment plans.

But as you'll discover in this chapter, this duality represents not just the progress but also the challenges inherent in healthcare technology. We'll explore why some technologies, as practical as EHR systems, still grapple with issues like usability and interoperability while others, like telemedicine, must navigate ethical and regulatory minefields.

The advent of AI in healthcare introduces a fresh set of questions, ethical conundrums, and logistical challenges.

Yet it also offers unprecedented opportunities for enhancing patient outcomes, streamlining operations, and even tackling previously untreatable conditions.

As we proceed, this chapter will leave you with a comprehensive understanding of the state of healthcare technology. You will gain insights into its current capabilities, its limitations, and the manifold possibilities that the future holds—especially with the integration of AI.

So, are you ready to explore the digital lifelines of healthcare, the technologies that are saving lives today, and those that promise to revolutionize our tomorrow? Let's dive in.

Current Healthcare Technology

Medical experts utilize a range of technologies, such as X-rays, MRIs, and a plethora of lab testing devices. These tools are essential for making precise patient diagnoses.

Artificial intelligence assists in medical imaging by detecting minor fractures, identifying tumors, and pinpointing areas of bleeding, among other tasks. Trained medical professionals rely on such technology to diagnose and treat millions of patients each year. The pace of technological advancement has been particularly rapid in the last half-decade. Here are some examples:

- **DNA genome research.** Genomic research in DNA can flag potential diseases or conditions before any symptoms manifest in a patient. Early identification allows for more timely treatment. Looking ahead, there may be possibilities to either repair or inhibit faulty DNA.

- **Ultra Sound.** For years, medical applications of sound waves have ranged from imaging to targeting and eliminating certain cancerous tumors to enhancing brain function.

- **Wearables.** Technological advancements in wearables like fitness trackers and smart rings offer valuable tools for tracking medical conditions like hypertension, breathing issues, and irregular heartbeats. These devices are particularly useful for keeping an eye on at-risk populations, including infants, seniors, individuals with chronic illnesses, and those with specific disabilities.

- **Robotics.** Robotics in the operating room is becoming the standard of care to assist surgeons in using smaller incision lines, causing less damage to normal tissue. Precision robotics provide improved outcomes for brain, spine, and thoracic surgeries.

- **MRNA technology.** mRNA technology may have gained popularity during the Covid-19 pandemic, but the technology has been improving over the past decade. It uses messenger ribonucleic acid (mRNA) to transport lab-generated genetic data into human cells.

- **Neurotech.** Devices designed to observe and evaluate brain activity can also deliver external stimuli to influence neural functions. One such device under development is the Neuralink brain implant.

Those are but a few of the innovations made in the last five years, and many more are being researched. The large-scale adoption and implementation of these technologies is justifiably slow in the medical field, yet it is progressing regardless.

A significant emphasis in the expansion and advancement of medical technology is geared toward providing patients with access to their health data, as actionable medical information can guide individuals in making lifestyle adjustments.

The Rise of AI in Healthcare

What Exactly Is AI?

Before we embark on discussing how AI is shaping healthcare, it's crucial to understand what AI means. According to McKinsey (2023), AI refers to "software or hardware that is designed to mimic human capabilities of sensing, comprehending, acting, and learning." Within AI, there are more specific categories, such as Applied AI, which pertains to systems that are designed to handle specific tasks (like diagnosing diseases), and Machine Learning, a subset of AI where the system learns from data rather than following pre-programmed rules.

Artificial Intelligence, as defined by McCarthy (2007), is "the science and engineering of making intelligent machines, especially intelligent computer programs. It is related to the similar task of using computers to understand human intelligence, but AI does not have to confine itself to methods that are biologically observable" (IBM, 2023).

Machine learning falls under the umbrella of artificial intelligence and computer science, with a focus on leveraging data and algorithms to replicate human learning processes and incrementally enhance accuracy. The algorithms analyze data and then create their own set of criteria through which that data is identifiable and manipulable. (IBM, 2023b)

AI Technology Accessibility

AI isn't a new concept; its roots trace back to the mid-20th century and to the work of British Mathematician, computer scientist, and logician Alna Turning. However, what's changed dramatically in recent years is the accessibility and awareness of AI technologies. In the past, AI was largely the domain of specialized research institutions and corporate giants with immense resources. Today, owing to advancements in affordable consumer hardware and the prevalence of cloud computing, AI tools and platforms have become available to the public, thereby equalizing access to this potent technology.

Though it's well-recognized that machines surpass humans in computational abilities, the degree of advancement in machine capabilities has been staggering. Several computers have now surpassed the exascale threshold, signifying their ability to execute quintillion computations every second. To put it in perspective, such a machine could accomplish more calculations in a single second than a highly intelligent human could in 31.5 billion years.

Real-World Examples of Accessible AI

To highlight the broad accessibility of AI, let's look at a few examples of free or widely available programs that are transforming different sectors:

- ChatGPT was designed by OpenAI with GPT (Generative Pre-trained Transformer) architecture. It was designed to be a conversational service. The current version, as of the last training data in 2022, is built on GPT-4, a large-scale machine learning model trained to predict the next word in a sequence of words. GPT-4 possesses 175 billion machine learning parameters, enabling it to produce text that resembles human writing, based on its training data. The success of ChatGPT is rooted in the fact that the generated text has a human-esque tone, closely mimicking real human speech and conversation (Sedinkina, 2023).

- ChatGPT is engineered to help with various tasks such as responding to queries, offering clarifications, creating text, and participating in discussions. It has applications in customer service, tutoring, content creation, and more. While the technology is advanced and can perform many tasks at a level that seems human-like, it's important to note that it lacks true understanding, consciousness, or emotions.

The model is trained on a diverse range of internet text but doesn't have the ability to access real-time information, browse the internet, or understand context beyond the text input it receives. It is not a specialized expert but a generalist model capable of discussing a wide array of topics.

OpenAI has successfully released versions of GPT, each with improvements in scale and performance, and the technology continues to be a subject of active research and development. Chat GPT has garnered attention for its versatility and user-friendliness.

- Midjourney is an advanced generative artificial intelligence program and service, developed and maintained by the independent research lab Midjourney, Inc., based in San Francisco. It generates images from natural language descriptions, called prompts, like OpenAI's DALL-E and Stability AI's Stable Diffusion. The tool is currently in open beta, which it entered on July 12, 2021.

- Currently, Midjourney is exclusively accessible through a Discord bot on its official Discord server. You can interact with it by directly messaging the bot or inviting the bot to a third-party server. Users "create" artwork with Midjourney using Discord bot commands . To generate images, users use the /imagine command and type in a prompt; the bot then returns a set of four images. From there, the images can be enhanced or modified. Further tweaks can be made to the prompt to help refine the produced images. David Holz is leading the team responsible for Midjourney. He is a co-founder of Leap Motion. In an August 2022 interview with The Register, Holz disclosed that the company had already achieved profitability. (Claburn, 2022)

- Visily is an AI-powered wireframe tool capable of swiftly converting screenshots, templates, or text prompts into modifiable wireframes and prototypes. Tailored for non-designers, it garners trust from a vast array of product managers, founders, developers, and business analysts. Visily boasts an intuitive interface, a comprehensive UI library, and enhanced AI functionalities, which collectively have expedited the discovery process for numerous companies substantially. It has helped distinguish good ideas from bad ones and simplified communication for teams. Visily is also capable of auto-populating labels, names, numbers, and images to save time. The tool is free to sign up for and does not require a credit card. Visily is loved by many companies such as Rewst, Swept Janitorial Software, PayBIX, interviewing.io, and SenseHawk. (Visily, 2023)

- Bing, a web search engine, is owned and managed by Microsoft. It offers an array of search services such as web, video, image, and map search functionalities. It is developed using ASP.NET. Microsoft has also integrated artificial intelligence into Bing to enhance its capabilities. Some of the features and capabilities are

Bing Chat: A conversational agent that can answer questions, provide explanations, generate text, and engage in conversation. It can also create images from natural language descriptions, called prompts.

Bing Summary: A feature that can summarize the content of web pages, books, articles, and other documents. It can also generate key takeaways and compare different sources of information.

Bing Translate: A feature capable of converting text and speech among various languages. It can also detect the language of the input and provide alternative translations.

- **Bing Content:** A feature that can help users create and improve their own content, such as poems, stories, emails, tweets, and more. It can also add humor, brevity, formality, and other styles to the text.

- **Bing Context:** A feature that allows users to access Bing Chat from the Edge Sidebar and use the current web page as a source of information. It can also keep the context of previous questions and provide more relevant answers.

The Influence and Future of AI

The rise of artificial intelligence is at a critical turning point in the annals of human invention, exerting an irreversible influence on myriad sectors—from healthcare and education to transportation and commerce. This groundbreaking technology carries with it an almost incomprehensible potential for catalyzing positive societal and economic transformations. For instance, in the realm of healthcare, AI can assist in data management and diagnostic accuracy, develop personalized treatment plans, and even predict the likelihood of certain diseases long before symptoms manifest. Similarly, in transportation, the advent of autonomous vehicles promises to enhance safety while reducing environmental impact. However, technology is not without its complexities and ethical implications.

It is imperative that we approach AI with both cautious optimism and critical awareness, particularly in domains where human lives are directly affected. Take healthcare as a pertinent example: AI-powered diagnostics and treatment options can revolutionize medicine. However, improper or irresponsible use could lead to catastrophic errors, highlighting the need for rigorous testing, measured and controlled deployments, and the imposition of necessary ethical boundaries.

Ultimately, as we stand on the cusp of a future increasingly influenced by AI, technology presents us with both unparalleled opportunities and serious ethical dilemmas. Balancing these two facets—optimizing and successfully exploiting the enormous potential for social good while diligently mitigating risks—is essential for the responsible evolution and deployment of Artificial Intelligence.

Implications of AI for Healthcare

Artificial intelligence has the potential to revolutionize various aspects of healthcare, offering both opportunities and challenges. Below are some of the key implications.

- **Improved Diagnostics.** AI algorithms can analyze medical images, genomic sequences, and other data to help identify diseases more quickly and accurately than human professionals.

- **Personalized Treatment.** AI can evaluate a patient's medical history, genetic composition, and additional factors to suggest treatment plans that are highly customized.

- **Predictive Analytics.** AI can predict outbreaks of infectious diseases, patient admission rates, and other important phenomena, allowing for better resource allocation.

- **Telemedicine and Remote Monitoring.** AI-powered systems can facilitate remote healthcare delivery, which is especially useful in rural or underserved areas.

- **Drug Discovery.** AI algorithms are capable of scrutinizing extensive datasets to foresee the interactions between various drugs and their targets, considerably accelerating the drug discovery process.

- **Efficiency and Cost-Effectiveness.** One of the immediate impacts of AI is the automation of repetitive tasks. Mundane but essential duties like data entry or appointment scheduling could be fully automated, freeing healthcare professionals to focus on more complex tasks that require human judgment.

- **Enhanced Surgical Procedures.** Robotics powered by AI can assist surgeons and even carry out specific tasks autonomously during surgeries.

- **Affordability and Accessibility.** By automating various processes, healthcare could become more cost-effective, which in turn could make it more accessible to wider populations.

- **Quality of Care.** Far from rendering human expertise obsolete, AI acts as a tool that can help health professionals perform better at their jobs, enhancing diagnosis accuracy and personalized treatment plans, thus improving outcomes for patients.

- **Expanding the Scope.** AI's current applications include but are not limited to disease diagnostics, personalized treatments, and even gene editing. These topics will be explored more thoroughly later in the book.

Transforming the Healthcare Landscape

The most significant promise that AI holds for healthcare is a transformative shift in clinical workflows. As outlined by Insider Intelligence (2023), AI can add immense value by automating or augmenting most of the tasks performed by clinicians and staff, thereby making healthcare delivery faster, more accurate, and more efficient. The scope of its application is diverse and far-reaching, covering both visual and physical domains.

- **Visual AI:** This includes tasks such as managing electronic medical records, streamlining outpatient appointments, and tracking patient health through various applications.

- **Physical AI:** Here, the impact is even more tactile, involving robotic surgeries, automated drug dispensing systems, and other mechanical tasks traditionally performed by human hands. (Shuaib et al., 2020).

Deep learning

A form of Machine Learning capable of processing not just plain text but also more complex data types like images and videos, often with minimal human intervention.

The foundation for deep learning lies in the human brain's neural network, which serves as the model for arranging the neural networks in deep learning programs. As these machine-based neural networks consume more data, they are designed to progressively learn and identify increasingly complex aspects of the data they process.

As it processes data, the model can form hypotheses about the information it's analyzing and then refine its understanding based on the accuracy of these hypotheses. This recurrent learning becomes another dataset that can help the model make fresh observations about new data or inform other models for future predictions. Different kinds of deep learning neural networks include:

- Feed-Forward Neural Networks: These represent the most basic type of neural networks, where data travels in one direction only, moving continuously from the input layer directly to the output layer without looping back to previous data. The network is "trained" to analyze specific datasets so that it can later apply that knowledge to new, unfamiliar datasets. These types of neural networks are most employed in the banking industry for identifying fraudulent transactions. The initial training involves feeding the AI a dataset where fraudulent transactions are tagged while legitimate ones are not. The AI then leverages this foundational understanding to spot patterns in new transactions, aiding in the detection of fraud.

- **Traditional Neural Networks (CNR).** Modeled after the animal visual cortex, these networks excel at perceptual tasks similar to those their biological counterparts handle. They are particularly effective at processing images and recognizing elements within those pictures. Applications range from identifying brand logos in photos to recognizing animal species from images or even analyzing medical scans for diagnoses. Initially, the network is trained with images containing a specific subject, allowing it to identify the unique traits of that subject—like the distinctive wing pattern, beak length, or foot type of a bird. Once trained, the network can then identify those traits in new images by seeking those specific characteristics.

- Recurrent Neural Networks (RNN): Contrary to feed-forward networks, these networks permit data to circulate in both forward and backward directions. They reintroduce old data alongside new inputs, providing the system with a sense of temporal context. This is particularly useful for processing text and images. While they can perform tasks like those of feed-forward networks, they do so in a more nuanced manner due to their capacity to recognize specific patterns.

In a banking context, both feed-forward and RNN systems can detect fraudulent activities. However, RNNs can also learn from an individual's general financial behaviors as though they have a memory. When new transactions occur, RNNs compare them to the individual's past financial history. For example, if client A has never made a transaction exceeding $1,000 in a five-year span but suddenly makes two such transactions within three days, the system can flag this as potentially fraudulent due to the significant deviation from typical activity.

Deep Learning is one of the more important AI and Machine Learning subtypes that will be used in healthcare. A customized, medical version of it will be the basis of the analytical and data processing systems used for AI diagnostic assistance and personalized treatment recommendations.

The Future Awaits: An AI-Integrated Healthcare System

Imagine a healthcare system where AI plays a pivotal role in every aspect:

- A primary care appointment where an AI-powered virtual assistant initially gathers patient data, medical history, and current symptoms, enabling the doctor to spend more time on diagnosis and treatment.

- In hospitals, robotic arms assist surgeons with high-precision tasks, minimizing human error and increasing the overall safety of difficult procedures. The added surgical precision creates less tissue damage, and patients experience shorter recovery times.

- AI algorithms sift through all available and pertinent medical literature to suggest the most current and effective treatments for various diseases, personalized to each patient's genetic makeup. Achieved through complex simulation of each potential treatment's interaction with the unique biology/genetics of each patient to find the optimal result.

By incorporating AI into these aspects and more, healthcare could transform into a system that is not just faster and more efficient but also more precise and personalized.

AI has the potential to redefine healthcare by automating mundane tasks, improving the quality of care, and even expanding the horizons of what's medically possible. The use of AI in healthcare is poised for exponential growth, bringing forth opportunities and challenges that we can scarcely imagine.

What Lies Ahead

Now that we've taken a comprehensive look at the dynamic landscape of current healthcare technology, it's crucial to examine the other side of the coin. The next chapter will investigate the potential that AI has to enhance the utility of existing medical technology and personnel. This critical exploration will help us better understand the immeasurable value and urgent necessity of AI integration in healthcare while also granting an appreciation for the justified caution needed in this endeavor. Are you ready to bridge the gap between what is and what could be?

Chapter 2:

Expanding the Horizons: The Untapped Potential of AI in Healthcare

In today's rapidly evolving healthcare landscape, traditional models are increasingly showing their limitations, whether it's the constraints of existing and approved technology or the pressure on overworked healthcare professionals. While these challenges persist, the advent of artificial intelligence offers a unique opportunity for all-encompassing transformative change. This chapter will discuss the specific shortcomings of our current healthcare systems, from outdated technology to over-stretched human resources, and demonstrate how AI technologies can provide innovative solutions to these pressing issues. By shedding light on the capability of AI to address these gaps, we provide a compelling foundation for the argument in favor of integrating AI into healthcare systems, not as a replacement but as a powerful adjunct that can drive more efficient, effective, and equitable care.

Imagine a world where epilepsy patients are not bound by the unpredictability of their next seizure but can live a life of relative certainty and safety. According to the World Health Organization's (WHO) 2023 report, over 50 million people suffer from epilepsy, and as many as 70% of these cases could be effectively managed to an asymptomatic level with the right diagnosis and treatment. The key issue for many epilepsy patients is the vagueness of most diagnoses, which often doesn't allow for a targeted, single-course treatment.

Professor Patrick Kwan and his team at Monash University are working on an AI model that offers a glimmer of hope for epilepsy patients (Hakeem et al., 2022). They are developing an AI algorithm that optimizes medication regimens for epilepsy patients, with the intended overarching goal being to assist patients in achieving seizure-free lives. Kwan points out that if patients are prescribed the wrong medication, they not only continue to experience seizures but may also suffer from side effects. "So, they're not gaining any benefit, but are actually being harmed by the medication," he says. The AI model evaluates a multitude of factors that would take a human an impractical amount of time to process. It's not just a futuristic vision; it's on the verge of becoming a reality.

The AI model was developed using medical data from several thousand patients across Australia, Malaysia, China, and the UK under the leadership of Associate Professor Zongyuan Ge (Hakeem et al., 2022). "It's truly exciting to observe how the newest deep learning models are extending their capabilities from aiding in diagnosis to actually informing treatment options," said Associate Professor Ge.

Case Studies in AI and Healthcare

RIKEN Center for Biosystems Dynamics Research (BDR) is a leading scientific research institute in Japan that focuses on understanding the principles governing dynamic biological systems. Situated at the intersection of various scientific disciplines like biology, physics, and computational science, BDR aims to shed light on the fundamental processes that govern life, from cellular mechanisms to whole-organism development. The center employs cutting-edge technologies and methodologies, including high-resolution imaging, bioinformatics, and other specialized techniques. Their work has significant implications not only for scientific understanding but also for practical applications, such as regenerative medicine and drug development. The center often collaborates with international partners to accelerate scientific discoveries and their translation into real-world solutions.

Verge Genomics is a biotechnology company that accelerates drug discovery by leveraging the power of machine learning and computational biology. The company focuses on understanding complex diseases at the genomic level, particularly those affecting the human brain, such as Alzheimer's, Parkinson's, and ALS. By analyzing vast datasets that include genetic information, Verge Genomics identifies promising drug targets and develops them more efficiently than companies that use traditional methods. Their innovative approach combines big data analysis with advanced algorithms, reducing the time and cost associated with drug discovery. The work done by Verge Genomics holds the potential to revolutionize the treatment of some of the most challenging and devastating diseases affecting humanity.

Nuance is a Microsoft company that offers technology solutions that are freeing up time for healthcare providers and enhancing the trust they share with their patients. Building and sustaining patient trust is crucial and is achieved through meaningful interactions—taking the time to listen, understand concerns, and provide thorough answers. Understanding the patient's verbal and non-verbal cues is vital for developing a tailored care plan, especially in primary care settings where long-term relationships are the cornerstone. Over time, these relationships can grow into strong emotional bonds, featuring moments of empathy and emotional support, which contribute to high-quality healthcare.

BotMD is a healthcare technology company specializing in AI-powered solutions designed to assist healthcare professionals. Their flagship product is an AI chatbot that functions as a clinical assistant, providing quick and accurate answers to medical queries. This tool eases the workload of healthcare workers by delivering instant access to clinical information, ranging from drug interactions and treatment guidelines to diagnostic criteria. Developed in collaboration with medical experts, BotMD's platform streamlines hospital workflows and enhances patient care by reducing the time clinicians spend on information retrieval, allowing them to focus more on patient interactions. Through its innovative use of AI, BotMD addresses critical challenges in healthcare, offering a scalable solution to improve efficiency and accuracy.

AI-driven technologies are aiding healthcare providers in offering superior care by minimizing administrative tasks. For example, primary care providers at the University of Michigan Health-West are leveraging mobile devices equipped with ambient listening to automatically record patient interactions and input data into the Health Records (Spiegel, 2023). This allows providers to concentrate on the patient rather than on data entry. Similarly, Fisher-Titus Medical Center employs workflow and documentation tools aimed at reducing administrative workload for doctors, making more time for patient interaction (Nuance, 2023). These technological solutions are not only enhancing work-life balance for clinicians but are also receiving positive feedback from patients, who find their healthcare providers more engaged and approachable.

As mentioned in Chapter 1, IBM's Watson has made notable strides in the healthcare sector, leveraging its advanced artificial intelligence capabilities to assist in various medical domains (IBM Education, 2023). Watson has been instrumental in oncology, helping doctors identify relevant treatments for cancer patients by analyzing medical records and vast volumes of scientific literature. It has also ventured into drug discovery, contributing to research efforts by sifting through complex biochemical data. Additionally, Watson has played a role in personalized medicine, aiding in the development of treatment plans tailored to individual genetic profiles. It has also been employed in administrative tasks to optimize hospital operations. While not without its challenges and limitations, IBM Watson has showcased the potential of AI in augmenting healthcare practices and advancing medical research.

While the success stories surrounding the application of AI in healthcare are indeed promising and inspiring, they represent just the tip of the iceberg when it comes to the technology's untapped potential. Having witnessed the transformative impact of AI in areas like diagnostics, treatment planning, and administrative efficiency, it's clear that we are on the cusp of a new frontier. Yet, beyond these well-documented achievements lies a vast expanse of possibilities still awaiting exploration. From revolutionizing preventive care to equalizing healthcare access globally, the prospective applications of AI are both numerous and profound. As we transition from celebrating the accomplishments to envisioning what's next, let's explore the uncharted territory of AI's potential to redefine healthcare as we know it.

The Untapped Potential of AI in Healthcare

The healthcare sector has been one of human civilization's most extraordinary accomplishments. From the discovery of antibiotics to the development of advanced surgical techniques, industry has continually redefined the limits of what's medically possible. Yet, even as we admire these strides, it's crucial to acknowledge that both healthcare technology and healthcare personnel—doctors, nurses, lab technicians, and others—face ongoing challenges.

The Limits of Current Healthcare Technology

The Complexity of Data Sharing and Collaboration in Healthcare

Among the myriad challenges facing healthcare today, the fragmented nature of healthcare data stands as one of the most urgent issues to address. At present, the exchange of vital healthcare data between different providers is characterized by a lack of consistency, leading to inefficient and often disjointed care. This gap in effective data sharing results not only in preventable operational difficulties but also in significant negative consequences for patients. The consequences range from delays in treatment to potentially harmful medical errors. According to an article in Forbes, advanced technology holds the key to significantly enhancing data interoperability, stating that leveraging these advancements is "critical" to improving access to care and elevating the healthcare industry for the benefit of both health systems and patients (Capone, 2022). The current failure in data coordination undermines the goals of comprehensive, timely, and efficient patient care, making the push for technological solutions to facilitate better data sharing essential for the next developmental stage in the modern healthcare landscape.

Initial Error Rates in Technology Adoption

One significant hurdle hindering the adoption of new technologies within healthcare settings is the issue of initial error rates. When a new system is implemented, it is often accompanied by glitches, inaccuracies, or other operational errors that can take time to identify and rectify. Even though these problems might be temporary and solvable, their very presence can serve as a major deterrent to embracing cutting-edge healthcare solutions.

An article in Physicians Practice underscores this by stating that the greatest challenge faced by the healthcare industry in adopting new technology is the high rate of initial errors (Boxler, 2020). This creates a ripple effect of hesitancy among healthcare providers, who may be cautious about introducing a new system that could disrupt patient care, even temporarily. As a result, this initial unreliability can significantly slow down technological advancement in healthcare, preventing the timely implementation of solutions that could otherwise improve both the efficiency and effectiveness of patient care.

This issue defies solving. The hesitancy from industry stakeholders and healthcare providers is justified. Their first obligation is to their patients, to protect the public and prioritize their health and wellbeing over potential technological advancements. When in their infancy, these new technologies can represent a minor threat to users, as is the nature of first generation or prototypes of machines. This can often stem from unrefined and unproven technology, even if that technology ultimately improves the healthcare landscape.

Financial Obstacles and Inequity in Healthcare Access

The march of technological progress in healthcare, while undoubtedly beneficial, often carries with it substantial financial costs. These costs can pose a formidable barrier to entry, particularly for patients who are underinsured or completely uninsured. As advanced diagnostic equipment, specialized treatments, and state-of-the-art medical facilities become increasingly integrated into standard care practices, the financial burden associated with accessing these resources can be prohibitive for many.

This economic hurdle serves to deepen one of the most pressing and persistent issues in healthcare: the glaring disparity in the quality of care accessible to different socioeconomic groups. Consequently, while advancements in medical technology have the potential to improve healthcare outcomes, their high costs risk widening the chasm between those who can afford top-tier medical services and those who are relegated to less effective or even substandard care options. In this way, the financial barriers linked with technological progress risk perpetuating, if not exacerbating, existing inequalities within the healthcare system.

The financial burden affects Hospitals also. The cost of purchasing, operating, and maintaining this cutting-edge technology is immense and is usually then passed onto the patient. It is why smaller hospitals in more remote areas, or those in underfunded/underdeveloped communities, tend to be significantly less well-equipped when compared to larger, wealthier institutions in bigger cities and developed nations. All patients, regardless of their location, deserve the same quality of care as those in more developed areas.

Additional Considerations

Further investigations into the complexities faced by hospital management reveal a gamut of issues, including entrenched bureaucratic systems, a lack of specialized administrative staff, and a general resistance to change among personnel. One glaring issue is the misalignment between current data-entry practices and the dynamic nature of a physician's daily responsibilities. Doctors often find themselves tethered to a computer terminal for inordinate amounts of time, entering data or navigating electronic health records. This practice is not only time-consuming but also incongruent with the fast-paced environment in which healthcare professionals operate. Such inefficiencies divert valuable time and attention away from direct patient care, exacerbating stress levels among medical staff and potentially impacting the quality of healthcare delivery.

The Human Element: A Double-Edged Sword

Human healthcare professionals, despite their exceptional skill and dedication, are not infallible. They can make mistakes or overlook details, leading to medical errors or delayed treatments. This is not just unfair to the patients who deserve optimal care but also to healthcare providers who are already stretched thin and are expected to operate without error perpetually. Healthcare professionals are humans with limitations, both physical and cognitive, that need acknowledgment and respect.

Let's be clear: Acknowledging limitations isn't the same as disregarding the colossal advancements that have been made in healthcare. Instead, it serves to highlight the incredible opportunity that exists for AI to come alongside current systems and personnel, augmenting their capabilities and minimizing their limitations. Progress and improvements have been made, yet it is essential to embrace the potential for an even better and more effective healthcare system. It is an ethical obligation for the healthcare sector to always continually pursue the improvement and enhancement of the healthcare experience for the public.

Artificial Intelligence can facilitate seamless data sharing, reduce initial error rates through robust testing and simulations, equalize access to healthcare by automating and optimizing processes, and reduce the administrative burden on healthcare professionals. These advancements can make healthcare safer, more efficient, and more equitable, all while respecting the human element at the heart of the industry.

So far, this chapter has established that while we have come far, there is still much to be done, and AI provides an extraordinary opportunity to do it. The following section will examine the ethical and societal considerations that come with these technological advancements.

Understanding Human Limitations in Healthcare

The Fallibility Factor

Human error is a variable that cannot be completely eliminated. The old adage, "To err is human," captures an essential truth. No matter the level of training or years of experience, healthcare providers—be they doctors, nurses, or lab technicians—make mistakes. According to a paper in the National Library of Medicine, healthcare providers are humans first, prone to the same lapses in judgment or focus that all humans experience (Dubeck, 2014).

The Fatigue Factor

Humans also get tired. Long hours, emotional stress, and the sheer mental focus required for medical work contribute to fatigue, which in turn increases the likelihood of error. Psychology Today highlights the need to impose reasonable limits on resident physicians' working hours (Breus 2011). Even if some surgeons manage to perform back-to-back 10-hour surgeries, it's generally not recommended due to the heightened risk of complications. This does not only relate to physicians, however. Even nurses and lab technicians need the same consideration. Overworked and stressed humans are known to make preventable errors (Marano 2020).

The Time Constraint Factor

Time is a finite resource. Each of us has exactly 24 hours in a day, no more, no less. The allocation of this time among various tasks, emergencies, and responsibilities puts immense pressure on healthcare providers. Forbes notes that physicians are often overloaded with administrative duties, leaving less time for patient care (Wu, 2019). Strategies to reduce the non-essential tasks of healthcare professionals should be developed and implemented promptly.

The Locality Factor

Healthcare professionals are bound to physical locations. While telemedicine has extended their reach somewhat, they still cannot be in multiple places at once. For instance, a doctor can't simultaneously perform surgery in one hospital while consulting in another, leading to service gaps that can be detrimental to patient care. Certain specialties are rare or understaffed. Currently, there are entire African and Asian cities that have no Oncologists or Pediatricians, and so have to request specialist physicians from a different city/country that may not always be available. (Khan & Raza, 2021; Miseda et al., 2017).

Additional Resources and Opinions

An article on **Forbes Tech Council** discusses how machine learning is addressing some of these human limitations.

A piece on **UHC Solutions** questions the number of patients a single physician can reasonably treat.

A **Medium** blog post discusses the unreasonable expectations often placed on healthcare providers, treating them as if they are infallible gods rather than humans.

<u>**Kevin MD**</u> emphasizes that physicians have their limits too, both professionally and personally, and should be respected as such.

Bringing It All Together: The AI Solution

In summarizing the limits of both modern healthcare technology and personnel, it becomes increasingly evident that the next step forward lies in the intersection of healthcare and AI. Artificial Intelligence offers scalable, sustainable solutions to these challenges:

Reducing Human Error. AI can assist in diagnostics, drug delivery, and treatment plans, thereby minimizing the scope of human error.

Combatting Fatigue. AI can handle routine tasks, freeing healthcare providers from administrative burdens and enabling them to focus more on patient care.

Optimizing Time. AI systems can manage appointments, keep track of patient history, and even provide initial screenings, making the most out of the limited time healthcare professionals have.

Overcoming Locality. Through telemedicine and, more importantly, remote monitoring, AI can extend the reach of healthcare providers, making quality healthcare accessible even in remote locations. A pertinent development in space is Telesurgery/Remote Surgery. This technology allows a physician, using robotics, to conduct surgery from a separate location. While still in its infancy, it can be integrated with artificial intelligence and help alleviate the local burden medical professionals have. A doctor in Toronto, Canada, can perform surgery on a patient in Arizona, USA.

Healthcare providers are incredibly skilled and dedicated but are limited by human constraints like fallibility, fatigue, time, and physical location. These limitations not only impact the quality of healthcare but also put unnecessary stress on medical professionals. Artificial intelligence provides an avenue to mitigate these limitations significantly, enabling healthcare to be more accurate, efficient, and accessible.

By understanding the boundaries of what both technology and humans can achieve in healthcare, we set the stage for a future where AI can augment these capabilities. The following chapters will explore this exciting frontier in greater detail, diving into specific use cases, ethical considerations, and the roadmap ahead.

Chapter 3

AI and Data Interoperability

The healthcare organizations that will be the most successful are the ones that will be able to fundamentally rethink and reimagine their workflows and processes and use machine learning and AI to create a truly intelligent health system. – (Marr, 2022)

Healthcare Data: The Challenge of Interoperability

Defining Interoperability in Healthcare

Interoperability refers to the ability of two or more disparate systems, applications, machines, or components to share crucial operational data with each other and for each unique system to interpret and make use of the exchanged data. Broadly speaking, it's the capacity for a diverse array of information systems, databases, applications, and tech devices to collaboratively share, swap, and access information. More pointedly, the data that is accessed must be comprehensible to all involved parties. To facilitate this, protocols are established, including the standardization of information formats and the implementation of translation packages.

Technical Interoperability

This level encompasses the fundamental infrastructure for data exchange, encompassing both hardware and software. For instance, achieving secure connectivity between a hospital's Electronic Health Record (EHR) system and a pharmacy's medication management system falls under technical interoperability. Elements such as connectors, data formats, and protocols (e.g., HL7 or FHIR) are integral to this aspect. Achieving this goal necessitates a collective industry effort to create and implement the required infrastructure.

Syntactic Interoperability

This deals with data structure and formats, making sure that the information can be read and interpreted at a basic level between systems. For instance, if one healthcare provider uses a PDF for medical records while another uses XML files, syntactic interoperability tools would translate between these different formats so that the data can be transferred and understood.

Semantic Interoperability

Semantic interoperability goes a step beyond and ensures that the meaning of the data remains consistent across different systems. For example, if one healthcare system records patient weight in kilograms and another in pounds, semantic interoperability would ensure that the receiving system understands the units of measurement and can convert them as necessary. This ensures that there is no misunderstanding of data that could lead to clinical errors. The creation of data translation keys involves designing a program that identifies the data's origin and applies necessary modifications to adapt it for its intended regional use—for example, an imperial to metric key and vice versa.

Organizational Interoperability

This encompasses the more intangible factors like governance, policy, and societal norms that impact how data is exchanged. An example could be the procedures, legislation, and policies that need to be in place to comply with laws such as the Health Insurance Portability and Accountability Act (HIPAA) in the United States, which ensures patient privacy. Additionally, it could involve developing common frameworks or governance structures that multiple organizations agree to adhere to for the purpose of efficient data exchange and collaboration.

By addressing these different layers of interoperability, healthcare systems can aspire to a seamless, efficient, and effective exchange of data, thus enhancing patient care.

Healthcare Workers Juggle Various Types of Data on a Daily Basis:

Electronic Health Records (EHRs):

Electronic Health Records are digital repositories of patient health information generated and maintained primarily by healthcare providers like hospitals and clinics. EHRs contain large amounts of data, including medical history, lab results, imaging studies, and medication records. They are instrumental for longitudinal patient care, enabling clinicians to have a more comprehensive view of a patient's health over time, thus facilitating more accurate diagnoses and personalized treatment plans.

Patient/Disease Registries:

Patient or disease registries are specialized databases that focus on collecting data about the incidence, prevalence, and treatment of specific diseases or medical conditions. These registries are often essential tools in epidemiological research, allowing scientists and healthcare professionals to monitor developing trends, evaluate outcomes, and identify potential areas for intervention or improvement. For instance, a cancer registry might track the efficacy of new treatments across a large patient population over time.

Health Surveys:

Health surveys usually originate from the general population and serve as a rich source of data on a range of public health issues. These surveys may address lifestyle factors, health behaviors, or disease prevalence, offering invaluable insights into the health status of a community or nation. The data collected can guide public health policies, help prioritize healthcare resource allocation, and serve as a foundation for further academic research.

Clinical Trials Data:

Data generated from clinical trials forms the backbone of medical research for new medications, therapies, and medical devices. Clinical trials involve controlled medical experiments designed to evaluate the effectiveness and safety of new treatments. The data collected is subjected to rigorous analysis and peer review and is a critical component in the approval process for new medications and medical procedures. Successful trials can lead to breakthroughs in treatment for diseases that currently have limited or ineffective options.

Additional types of data can include imaging data, lab results, and genetic information, all of which play pivotal roles in patient diagnosis and treatment.

Dependence on Interoperability in Modern Healthcare

The argument for implementing interoperability within healthcare settings is both timely and crucial. In an era where precision medicine is becoming the norm, having the *right* information accessible to the *right* healthcare provider at the *right* time isn't just a luxury; it's a necessity. A lack of interoperability can result in significant gaps in a patient's medical history, communication breakdowns between healthcare providers, and even severe medical risks like adverse drug interactions. For example, without interoperable systems, a specialist might not have immediate access to a patient's allergy information stored in a primary care physician's electronic health records, risking a dangerous or even fatal medical error. Additionally, having easy access to patient data, such as blood types in the trauma ward, can alleviate the constant need for universal donor O-negative blood. This is a crucial resource that needs conservation, and the available data helps mitigate the effects of a potential O-negative shortage.

Moreover, the importance of interoperability extends beyond the immediate sphere of patient care. Advancing the field of medical research is also affected. With the increasing importance of data-driven research methodologies, interoperable systems allow for more effective collection and analysis of real-world data. This is particularly relevant in the growing field of real-world evidence, where researchers analyze data from actual healthcare scenarios (as opposed to controlled clinical trials) to generate insights into drug effectiveness, treatment patterns, and patient outcomes. Interoperable data systems enable easier sharing and pooling of this kind of data across different institutions and studies, thereby enriching the quality of research and its potential impact on patient care.

Interoperability is not just a technical requirement but a fundamental building block for both optimizing patient care and accelerating medical research in the 21st century.

The Economic Aspect

The economic ramifications of lacking interoperability in healthcare are staggering. It is projected that administrative expenses account for more than one-third of the healthcare spending in the United States. These costs encompass billing complexities, manual data entry, insurance verification, and the complicated bureaucracy that often hampers efficient care delivery. The financial burden of these inefficiencies is not trivial; it significantly inflates the overall costs of healthcare, both for providers and patients.

According to some estimates, standardizing electronic healthcare information exchange could result in annual savings of up to $78 billion (NIH, 2020). This staggering sum could be redirected toward improving patient care, medical research, and healthcare infrastructure. The savings come from eliminating redundant tests, reducing administrative overhead, optimizing resource allocation, and enhancing preventive care through better data analytics. For example, if a patient's complete medical history is readily available across different healthcare providers, it could reduce the need for duplicate tests and procedures, thereby saving both time and money.

In a healthcare system that is often criticized for its inefficiency and high costs, the economic benefits of interoperability offer a compelling case for rapid adoption. By investing in interoperable systems, healthcare providers are not merely improving the quality and safety of patient care but are also taking a significant step toward a more economically sustainable model of healthcare delivery.

The Speed and Continuity Factor

In the fast-paced landscape of modern healthcare, speed and continuity are more than convenience; they are essential factors that can significantly influence patient outcomes. The ability to quickly and seamlessly transfer medical records, test results, and care plans across various healthcare providers and systems is crucial, especially in time-sensitive situations such as emergencies or acute medical conditions. For example, if a patient arrives at an emergency room experiencing severe allergic reactions, immediate access to their medical history can help clinicians make rapid, informed decisions about their treatment, thereby potentially saving their life.

Moreover, interoperability is not just critical during emergencies; it is equally important when a patient transitions from one healthcare system to another, perhaps due to relocation or a referral to a specialized medical center. In these scenarios, the smooth transfer of medical information ensures that the receiving healthcare provider has all the essential data to continue effective treatment without unnecessary delays or repetitions of very costly diagnostic tests. The continuity of care is thus maintained, reducing the likelihood of medical errors and enhancing the overall quality of healthcare delivery.

A recent University of Chicago Medicine study found that primary care clinicians would have to work 26.7 hours per day to accommodate recommended patient care (McPhee, 2022). Clinicians have indicated that they spend half of their day on administrative tasks, leaving only a quarter of their day for time in the exam room (AAFP, n.d.). Clinicians spend half of their exam room time having direct face-to-face interaction with patients, and nearly 40 percent entering or retrieving data on the computer.

Detailed clinical documentation is essential for providing quality care, but creating and accessing it can dominate clinicians' time, making patients feel like they are competing for attention.

Thus, the speed and continuity facilitated by interoperability are not just about operational efficiency; they are key elements that can substantially improve—and sometimes even save—lives. The case for healthcare interoperability is not merely a question of technology or economics but one of patient safety and the quality of medical care.

The Future of Healthcare, Data, and the Role of AI

The future landscape of healthcare is set to be shaped not merely by the sheer volume of data we collect but, critically, by how effectively that data is shared, analyzed, and utilized to improve patient care and healthcare systems. Accumulating data for its own sake is insufficient; the real value lies in its seamless integration and interoperable exchange across different platforms and healthcare providers. This is a perfect use for artificial intelligence. As we will explore in the chapters that follow, AI holds the potential to act as a transformative catalyst in achieving healthcare data interoperability on an unprecedented scale.

AI can enhance data management processes by making them more streamlined, efficient, and less susceptible to human errors. It can also analyze vast amounts of complex medical data at speeds incomprehensible to human clinicians, uncovering insights that can guide medical decisions and even predict health outcomes. By doing so, AI can make our healthcare systems not only more efficient but also significantly less costly.

However, the ultimate test of any advancement in healthcare technology is its effectiveness in saving lives and improving the quality of care. In this regard, AI shows immense promise. By facilitating more robust data sharing and utilization, AI has the potential to improve diagnostic accuracy, enhance truly personalized treatment plans, and even anticipate patient medical issues before they become life-threatening. On a larger scale, the AI can also predict more general health trends, such as disease outbreaks, aiding the medical sector in better preparedness.

The future of healthcare hinges on our ability to effectively leverage data. AI stands at the forefront of this endeavor, offering promising avenues for making healthcare more efficient, more cost-effective, and, most importantly, more effective at saving lives.

A prime example of the need for interoperability was the Covid-19 pandemic. Initially, all treatment trials and testing methods were being evaluated independently of each other. Early in the pandemic, data was scarce, and the limited information available was often not exchanged between institutions and nations. Time and resources were wasted, and lives lost that could have potentially been saved. More efficient data collection and sharing could have changed the course of the pandemic with earlier effective treatments developed and earlier widespread testing implemented. Vaccines and medications could have been developed sooner. Pharmaceutical companies also lamented the initial data shortage as it hampered their research and development of vaccines and drug treatments.

The Imperative for Interoperability: A View From the Patient's Lens

In the realm of healthcare, one of the most urgent and palpable problems is the inconsistent sharing of vital medical data among various healthcare providers. From the perspective of patients, this limitation is not merely an administrative hindrance but a matter that directly impacts their health and well-being. As highlighted in a Forbes article, the failure to routinely share healthcare data can create a domino effect of avoidable complications, including unnecessary delays in treatment, frustrations for both healthcare providers and patients, and, most concerning of all, potentially hazardous medical outcomes (Hayes, 2021).

Imagine, for instance, a patient with a complex medical history involving multiple specialists. If these specialists are unable to quickly and accurately share and access that patient's records, the risk for error—such as prescribing contraindicated medications or duplicating diagnostic tests—dramatically increases. Similarly, in emergency situations where every second counts, the absence of readily available medical history can delay life-saving treatments and may even result in fatal consequences.

The psychological stress experienced by patients should not be underestimated. Having to recount medical histories or facilitating the transfer of medical records between different providers can be time-consuming and stressful, detracting from the mental and emotional reserves a patient needs for healing and recovery.

Therefore, the call for data interoperability is not just an abstract, systemic issue; it's a deeply personal one. Every delay and every missing piece of information could mean a significant difference in the diagnosis, treatment, and, ultimately, the life of a patient. It is no exaggeration to say that enhancing data interoperability stands to dramatically improve not just the efficiency of healthcare systems but, more importantly, the quality and safety of patient care.

Streamlined Healthcare Experience

Imagine a healthcare journey devoid of redundant paperwork or the anxiety of waiting for crucial test results from another facility. Effective interoperability holds the promise of creating such a seamless experience. "In a 2018 survey of U.S. health system executives and finance leaders, 52% said that data sharing is the technology that will have the biggest positive impact on the patient experience" (Forbes, 2021).

These systems could alleviate logistical hassles, enabling patients to focus more on their recovery and less on administrative tasks.

Autonomy and Informed Decisions

Interoperability also heralds a new era of patient empowerment. With easier and more transparent access to their healthcare data, patients can actively participate in decision-making processes about their treatment plans. This increased level of autonomy allows patients to be better informed and more engaged in their healthcare journey, facilitating a more collaborative approach to care.

Enhanced Data Management

AI's data-processing capabilities are unparalleled. Not only can these algorithms sift through enormous datasets at speeds unimaginable to humans, but they can also summarize complex medical histories into easily digestible formats. For healthcare providers, this means having the critical information they require right at their fingertips, precisely when they need it the most.

Predictive Analysis

AI's capabilities extend beyond mere data presentation. Its sophisticated algorithms can analyze medical trends and patterns to predict future events, such as potential outbreaks or hospital readmissions. This predictive analysis adds a proactive element to healthcare, allowing healthcare systems to anticipate issues before they become crises, thereby substantially improving patient outcomes.

Patient-Centric Approach

AI's potential to personalize healthcare is groundbreaking. By processing and analyzing patient data from multiple sources, AI can produce individualized treatment recommendations that consider a full spectrum of factors, including medical histories and social determinants of health. This shift towards a more personalized, patient-centric model of care could revolutionize healthcare delivery.

Security

Data security is paramount in healthcare. AI can play a pivotal role in safeguarding sensitive patient information. Utilizing advanced encryption methods and cutting-edge anomaly detection techniques, AI can detect and prevent unauthorized data access. This adds extra security, keeping patient data confidential and secure.

For the average patient, interoperability may seem like a technical term that doesn't affect them directly. However, when fully realized, interoperability can revolutionize their healthcare experience, reducing inefficiencies, delays, and, most importantly, medical errors. As we move towards a future where healthcare data is both abundant and complex, the role of AI in streamlining interoperability becomes not just advantageous but essential. It's not an exaggeration to say that AI-driven interoperability has the potential to redefine the patient's experience, making healthcare more effective, efficient, and, above all, patient-centered.

The Contribution of Large Language Models to Healthcare Data Interoperability

Large Language Models (LLMs) are cultivated through extensive training on vast datasets that include billions of words. Their design enables them to comprehend, produce, and manipulate human language. As Forbes suggests, these LLMs are swiftly becoming a cornerstone in the future of healthcare data interoperability (Kuhn, 2023). But how do they fit into the larger ecosystem of healthcare?

Simplifying Complex Data

Healthcare data is often stored in unstructured formats like PDFs, handwritten notes, or transcribed voice recordings. Traditional databases find it challenging to parse this type of data. LLMs can excel here, understanding the context and content of unstructured data and converting it into a more structured, usable format.

Enhancing Semantic Understanding

LLMs can provide semantic understanding, a level of data interpretation that goes beyond mere keyword searches. This can be instrumental in complex cases where nuanced interpretation is required, adding a layer of depth to data analytics in healthcare.

Real-time Decision Support

LLMs can be integrated into Electronic Health Record (EHR) systems to offer real-time decision support to healthcare providers. They can analyze vast amounts of data instantly and provide evidence-based recommendations, thus reducing the cognitive load on medical personnel.

Natural Language Processing (NLP) and Interoperability

Natural Language Processing, a subfield of AI where LLMs play a significant role, is becoming crucial for healthcare data interoperability. It can convert human language data into machine-readable formats, providing seamless data exchange across different healthcare platforms. It can also assist in converting old non-digital (handwritten) or badly formatted data into standardized electronic records.

Data Interoperability & AI Advancement

Why AI is Essential

Achieving interoperability in healthcare data is a monumental task when done manually, riddled with the risk of errors, omissions, and delays. AI, particularly LLMs, can automate and streamline this process, allowing human resources to be redirected towards more patient-centric tasks like care and treatment.

For a machine learning algorithm to be effectively trained, it requires data that is both structured and well-formatted. Introducing poorly structured or incorrectly formatted data could lead to errors and distort the outcome of the analysis. This underscores the importance of adhering to standardized data formats and syntax.

For instance, if an AI is programmed to identify genetic anomalies related to diabetes, feeding it unstructured information could cause it to incorrectly flag individuals who don't actually have diabetes but do exhibit some of the specific biological results it's trained to look for. Such errors can distort the assignment's results and stray from the AI's intended parameters, making these mistakes difficult to spot in a dataset comprising millions of entries. Moreover, the datasets these AI are trained on need to be very diverse. This prevents the AI from developing a bias in its functionality. We will discuss AI bias in depth later on.

Human Effort vs. AI

While human expertise is irreplaceable in healthcare, the tedious task of managing data for interoperability can be offloaded to AI algorithms. This allows medical professionals to focus more on what they do best: diagnosing, treating, and caring for patients.

The Future is Interoperable and Intelligent

As we look toward the future, the importance of healthcare data interoperability cannot be overstated. Not only does it make the healthcare system more efficient and safer, but it also vastly improves the patient's experience. With the advent of sophisticated AI tools like Large Language Models, the dream of fully interoperable healthcare is closer than ever. AI holds the promise of transforming healthcare data management, freeing human resources to engage in more meaningful, high-value tasks, and ultimately providing better healthcare outcomes for all.

By embracing AI and LLMs, we're not just streamlining administrative procedures; we are transforming the healthcare delivery approach, enhancing its efficiency, personalization, and focus on patient needs.

Chapter 4

The Patient's Perspective

This chapter explores the prevalent concerns and issues that patients frequently raise about healthcare systems. It seeks to explore whether these issues can be resolved—or at least alleviated—through improved data interoperability and management aided by artificial intelligence.

"According to a systematic review of 59 studies involving 88,069 records, most patients complain about the management of their healthcare organization (35.1%). The second most-complained aspect is the safety and quality of the clinical care they received (33.7%), and the third highest is about the staff-patient experience they had (29.1%)" (Reader et al., 2014).

The System Isn't Perfect: Achievements and Shortcomings

Although healthcare systems have been instrumental in saving numerous lives and often function effectively for a large segment of the population, they are not without their flaws. A significant number of patients voice similar complaints and concerns, highlighting the presence of systemic issues that require urgent attention. From administrative inefficiencies to lapses in patient-centered care, these grievances point to areas where healthcare services can be improved to meet the needs of all patients more comprehensively.

Delays: A Persistent Issue Impacting Patient Care and Outcomes

Among the most frequent concerns expressed by patients is the issue of noticeable time delays in receiving timely medical care. Such delays manifest in various forms—ranging from extended waiting periods in emergency rooms to rescheduled surgeries and belated diagnoses. "Complaints highlight the impact that delays in care can have on people, both physically and psychologically, particularly where their health is deteriorating, and there is a lack of certainty about when care will be received," McDowell said (Radio New Zealand, 2023).

A report from the New Zealand health watchdog underscores that the consequences of these delays are a recurring subject in patient complaints (Impact of Delay, 2023). These aren't mere inconveniences; in rare instances, they can be matters of life and death. Delays in care can exacerbate existing health conditions, sometimes irreversibly, and create avoidable stress and uncertainty for patients and their families.

The reasons for delays in healthcare settings are multifaceted and complex. In emergency departments, for example, the most significant cause of delay is often the time delays between a patient's admission to the emergency room and their transfer to an available inpatient bed. This bottleneck isn't usually attributable to any single individual's shortcomings. Rather, it signifies a healthcare system that is operating beyond its capacity. In essence, extended wait times are less a fault of specific healthcare professionals and more a symptom of systemic inefficiencies and resource limitations.

Staff-Patient Relationship: A Significant Source of Patient Dissatisfaction

The staff-patient relationship ranks as the third most frequent subject of patient complaints, contributing to 29.1% of the issues raised. Patients commonly report instances of rudeness, indifference, or lack of empathy from healthcare staff, experiences that can substantially tarnish their overall healthcare journey and erode trust in the system.

The reasons behind such lapses in the staff-patient relationship are numerous and interconnected. Staff rudeness or inattentiveness may be symptomatic of deeper organizational issues such as long working hours, high stress levels, and a lack of emphasis on interpersonal training. These factors not only strain healthcare providers but also manifest as suboptimal patient care. Addressing these underlying challenges will be critical in improving both staff wellbeing and patient satisfaction.

Management Concerns: A Major Driver of Patient Complaints

A significant 35.1% of patient complaints are directed at the management of healthcare organizations (Reader et al., 2014). These complaints typically revolve around administrative and bureaucratic hurdles, such as convoluted procedures, excessive documentation requirements, and a prevailing lack of transparency in the system.

The root causes of these management-related complaints are often multifaceted. In many cases, they can be attributed to inefficient organizational systems and resource constraints. For example, poorly designed appointment allocation policies might result in unnecessarily long waiting times, even when the facility has the capacity to meet patient demand. Such systemic inefficiencies create a cycle of dissatisfaction and inefficiency that demands urgent attention.

The Underlying Flaws in the Healthcare System

To comprehend the root causes of the prevalent complaints in healthcare, it's essential to examine the intricate dynamics that govern the system's operation. These complaints are not isolated incidents but rather symptoms of deeper systemic issues that plague the healthcare landscape. A lack of adequate resources—be it staffing, equipment, or funding—often serves as a critical bottleneck, limiting the system's efficiency and effectiveness. Outdated technology further hampers the smooth functioning of healthcare services, resulting in process delays that impact both healthcare providers and patients. Additionally, insufficient training in both technical and interpersonal skills for healthcare professionals can lead to errors, miscommunications, and deteriorating staff-patient relationships. These multifaceted challenges cumulatively contribute to the shortcomings and grievances that many experience when interacting with healthcare systems.

Why Do Delays Happen?

Delays in healthcare settings are rarely attributable to a single factor; rather, they often arise from a complex interplay of systemic issues. A prime example is the bottleneck often encountered in emergency departments, where a lack of available beds in specialized units can create a cascading effect that prolongs patient wait times. But the issue doesn't stop there. Other contributing factors include staffing shortages, which can lead to overworked healthcare professionals being less capable of quick decision-making, systematic inefficiencies between various departments which mean patients are not handed over to relevant specialist departments as quickly as they otherwise could. It could also be outdated or incompatible technology, which hampers efficient data sharing and coordination among departments, or bureaucratic hurdles like insurance authorizations, which can add unnecessary layers of complexity.

Another cause of delays stems from resource limitations, such as dwindling or unavailable supplies of specific medications. Although these delays adversely affect patients, immediate solutions are often unfeasible. The same issue extends to medical equipment; in some regions, non-critical patients must schedule X-rays days in advance for a procedure that takes mere minutes.

Additionally, unexpected surges in patient volumes, sometimes due to seasonal illnesses or public health emergencies (like a pandemic), can strain the system even further. All these elements collectively contribute to delays, making them a stubborn challenge that defies easy or quick solutions.

Why Is There Mismanagement?

Mismanagement in healthcare can stem from a variety of factors, each contributing to less-than-optimal patient outcomes and systemic inefficiencies. Key issues often include poor allocation of resources, insufficient staffing, and outdated or incompatible technology systems that hamper effective communication and data sharing. Bureaucratic challenges, such as cumbersome paperwork and unclear protocols, can further complicate the delivery of care.

These managerial shortcomings can lead to long patient wait times, misdiagnoses, and even preventable medical errors. Moreover, when healthcare organizations are poorly managed, staff morale may suffer, exacerbating existing challenges and leading to a cyclical pattern of inefficiency and substandard care. Addressing these issues is critical not just for the well-being of patients but also for the overall health of the healthcare system.

Why Are Staff Sometimes Rude?

The instances of rudeness from healthcare staff are frequently the result of a combination of factors rather than individual ill-will. Often operating under high stress and prolonged work hours, healthcare professionals may find it challenging to maintain optimal levels of patient interaction. The demanding nature of their job can lead to emotional exhaustion and decreased patience, factors that could contribute to impolite or indifferent behavior. Additionally, medical training programs may prioritize clinical skills over interpersonal skills, leading to gaps in the ability to manage patient interactions effectively. All these factors can converge to create a situation where staff may come across as rude, affecting the patient's experience and overall trust in the healthcare system.

In the next sections, we will explore how AI and improved data management can potentially alleviate these systemic issues, thereby enhancing patient satisfaction and healthcare outcomes.

AI as a Solution

Artificial intelligence offers promising solutions to the healthcare sector's most pressing challenges, particularly in addressing patient complaints around delays, staff-patient relationships, and patient data management.

Addressing Delays Through AI

Artificial intelligence is increasingly playing a pivotal role in reducing delays within healthcare settings by optimizing hospital workflows. Various studies have demonstrated that the integration of AI-powered predictive analytics can significantly enhance patient flow, minimizing waiting times for consultations, tests, and treatments. For example, some hospitals have employed AI algorithms to predict patient admission rates, thereby efficiently allocating resources and staff. This technological intervention not only alleviates the stress on overburdened healthcare systems but also directly contributes to more timely and effective patient care.

AI not only expedites administrative tasks but also significantly reduces the time clinicians need to sift through medical histories and diagnostic results. Improved interoperability—made possible by AI—ensures that a patient's complete medical history is instantly available, thus streamlining the decision-making process.

Incorporating Interoperability for Reduced Wait Times: An Elaboration

Seamless data sharing through enhanced interoperability can have a transformative impact on healthcare efficiency, particularly in reducing patient wait times. A compelling study has indicated that improved interoperability could contribute to a remarkable 30-40% reduction in the time patients spend waiting for services (Tsai et al., 2020). This is because when healthcare providers have immediate access to patient records, diagnoses, and treatment plans from various platforms, they can make faster and more informed decisions. The efficient exchange of data can streamline the entire care delivery process, from initial consultation to final treatment. As a result, patients experience fewer delays, medical staff can allocate their time more effectively, and healthcare facilities can optimize their operational workflows. Improved interoperability thus stands as a powerful solution to one of healthcare's most pressing inefficiencies.

Enhancing the Staff-Patient Relationship through AI

The quality of the staff-patient relationship is a cornerstone of effective healthcare delivery, influencing not only patient satisfaction but also treatment outcomes. While concerns exist about the dehumanizing potential of technology, some experts propose that AI could serve to enrich these critical interactions. According to a study, the integration of AI into healthcare systems has the potential to remove repetitive and mundane tasks from clinicians, thereby allowing them to spend more meaningful time in direct patient engagement.

Take the example of AI-powered chatbots. These sophisticated algorithms can handle a multitude of administrative tasks that would otherwise consume the valuable time of medical staff. From answering routine questions and providing basic health advice to scheduling appointments and sending out treatment reminders, chatbots can significantly reduce the administrative burden on healthcare professionals.

This newfound freedom allows doctors, nurses, and other medical staff to channel their efforts more fully into direct patient care, fostering stronger relationships and ultimately enhancing the overall patient experience. Therefore, far from distancing healthcare providers from their patients, the smart application of AI can act as a facilitator for deeper, more meaningful interactions.

Interoperability and Personalized Care Enhanced by AI: A Comprehensive View

The role of AI in fostering interoperability reaches beyond simply streamlining administrative tasks or reducing wait times; it also has the potential to dramatically enhance the level of personalized care that healthcare professionals can offer. According to experts, AI has the capability to generate more detailed information about individual patients, including their optimal treatment paths and likely outcomes (Davenport & Kalakota, 2019). This type of data can profoundly impact the clinician-patient relationship by setting the stage for more meaningful shared decision-making.

"Additionally, AI might provide richer and more specific information about an individual patient's treatment options and expected outcomes. Such personalized data could allow clinicians to engage their patients more meaningfully in shared decision making" (Nagy & Sisk, 2020).

In a healthcare setting that is powered by AI and robust data interoperability, clinicians aren't merely operating with a snapshot of a patient's current condition. Instead, they have access to a comprehensive medical history, previous treatment responses, and even predictive analytics suggesting future health scenarios. This wealth of information, readily accessible thanks to seamless data sharing, allows healthcare providers to tailor their consultations, advice, and treatment plans to the specific needs and circumstances of each patient. As a result, medical interactions become less transactional and more substantive, with a focus on collaborative care planning. Patients are better informed and can participate more actively in their healthcare journey, leading to a more empowered patient base and, ultimately, better health outcomes.

Improving Patient Data Management Through AI and Interoperability

Issues surrounding the management of healthcare organizations are a significant source of patient dissatisfaction. These complaints often center around bureaucratic inefficiencies like data mismanagement, cumbersome billing processes, and complicated insurance claims. Advanced AI algorithms are poised to revolutionize this landscape by automating and optimizing these tasks, leading to more efficient and user-friendly healthcare systems. According to Healthcare IT News, AI is rapidly making strides in meeting complex data requirements and facilitating data interoperability, thereby transforming the very fabric of healthcare data management.

The Significance of Interoperability

When healthcare systems are well-integrated and interoperable, it elevates the entire experience for patients and healthcare providers alike. For example, a fully interoperable system enables real-time updates to patient records, which can be accessed quickly and efficiently by any authorized medical professional involved in the patient's care. This high level of integration negates the need for patients to fill out repetitive forms or provide the same information at different medical facilities. It also minimizes the risk of errors stemming from outdated or missing information. Ultimately, enhanced interoperability makes for a smoother, more straightforward, and less stressful experience for patients while allowing healthcare providers to deliver more accurate and timely care.

In summary, the three most common complaints in healthcare—delays, staff-patient relationships, and data management—highlight systemic inefficiencies that can be considerably improved with AI.

- **Delays:** AI can enhance workflows and facilitate instantaneous data sharing, thus minimizing waiting times.

- **Staff-Patient Relationships:** AI can take over routine tasks, allowing healthcare providers to focus more on patient interaction and personalized care.

- **Data Management:** AI brings efficiency and improved interoperability, streamlining administrative processes and thereby improving the patient's experience.

In the next chapter, we will discuss the practical applications and case studies that highlight how AI is already making a significant impact in addressing these challenges.

Chapter 5:

The Dawn of Personalized Healthcare: AI as a Catalyst

The foundation of personalized medicine rests on the emergence of new-fangled technology that is making certain diagnostic tests more affordable, accurate, and more in sync with overall patient care requirements.
– Morris Panner

In this chapter, we will examine the concept of personalized healthcare, exploring the need and demand for medical treatments tailored specifically for each patient and how AI can potentially improve and optimize these treatments.

The Dream of Personalized Healthcare

The idea of personalized healthcare—where medical treatments, diagnoses, and care plans are customized to each individual patient—has been a long-standing aspiration within the medical community. This vision goes beyond the standardized approach to offer targeted treatments that consider a person's genetic makeup, lifestyle, and even social determinants of health. However, the realization of this vision has been held back by various challenges, primarily technological limitations and the complexities inherent in managing vast and diverse sets of medical data.

In the past, even the most advanced healthcare systems struggled with the integration and analysis of different types of data, including electronic health records, genomic data, and real-world evidence from wearable devices. Compounding the issue is the diversity of data formats and the segregated nature of healthcare data repositories. All these factors together made it incredibly difficult to implement personalized healthcare solutions at scale.

Enter artificial intelligence. As a technology capable of analyzing huge data sets with a complexity far beyond human capability, AI is increasingly seen as the game-changer that could finally bring the concept of personalized healthcare to fruition. Not only can AI algorithms sift through and analyze extensive medical databases, but they can also learn from this data to predict patient outcomes, recommend personalized treatment plans, and even identify potential health issues before they become critical.

Machine learning models can analyze a patient's entire medical history, genetic data, lifestyle choices, and more to offer tailored recommendations that could range from personalized drug prescriptions to customized fitness plans. With AI, we are not moving into the era of personalized medicine; we are sprinting into it, breaking down the long-standing barriers that have kept this revolutionary approach from becoming a practical reality.

Enhancing the Human Element in Healthcare

The objective extends beyond the mere accuracy of medical treatments; it's about recognizing and treating patients as unique beings, each with their own specific health needs, aspirations, and goals. Modern healthcare is seeing a paradigm shift where patients are no longer passive recipients of medical care but active, informed partners in their healthcare journey. They want to be engaged at every level, from preventive measures to treatment decisions, underscoring the need for a healthcare approach that is not just clinically precise but also personally meaningful.

The Rising Demand

As genetic testing becomes more sophisticated and accessible, and as public awareness around personalized healthcare continues to soar, a powerful synergy is taking shape. This compelling combination is driving an unprecedented demand for healthcare solutions that are tailor-made for individual needs. No longer content to be passive participants in their health journeys, people are now seeking active roles, desiring treatments that consider their unique genetic makeup, lifestyle, and even personal preferences. This surge of interest is not just a fleeting trend but a significant shift, signaling the healthcare industry's move away from a standardized model towards an era of deeply personalized medical care.

Generational Preferences in Personalized Healthcare

The desire for personalized healthcare transcends generational boundaries, yet it manifests in distinct ways among different age groups, underscoring the complexity and dynamism of modern healthcare needs. Millennials, armed with technology and a penchant for convenience, often seek healthcare solutions that fit seamlessly into their digital lives (TRIARE, 2023). They want to consult with healthcare providers from the comfort of their homes, just as they would order dinner. On the flip side, baby boomers tend to value face-to-face interactions and have a more traditional approach, often prioritizing long-term relationships with primary care providers.

These contrasting preferences serve as a vivid reminder that personalized healthcare isn't solely about tailoring medical treatments to individual biological needs; it's also about adapting the mode and manner of healthcare delivery to align with the cultural and generational expectations of diverse patient populations.

The Complex Landscape of Personalized Healthcare Challenges

The prospect of personalized healthcare holds enormous promise, offering the potential for more effective treatments, improved patient outcomes, and a more efficient healthcare system. However, this optimistic vision is clouded by a series of significant challenges that stand in the way of its full realization. Among these hurdles are the high costs associated with personalized treatments, which can be prohibitive for both healthcare providers and patients. Additionally, there are complexities in resource allocation as the medical community grapples with how to most effectively deploy limited assets like specialized medical expertise, advanced diagnostic tools, and cutting-edge treatments.

Beyond financial and logistical concerns, there are also significant scientific obstacles. The empirical validation of personalized treatment regimens can be both time-consuming and expensive, requiring robust clinical trials and real-world evidence to establish their efficacy and safety. Ethical questions, too, abound—ranging from data privacy concerns to the equitable distribution of advanced treatments, which can risk exacerbating healthcare disparities.

Lastly, managing patient expectations adds another layer of complexity. In an age of instant information, patients are increasingly well-informed and have high expectations for personalized care, but the technology and methodologies to provide such care are still evolving and still have a way to go before they catch up with the idealized realities patients might have about what truly personalized healthcare is. All these challenges necessitate inventive, multi-disciplinary solutions to truly transform the healthcare landscape into one where personalized medicine isn't just a lofty ideal but a widespread reality.

Cost

The soaring costs associated with cutting-edge diagnostic tests and specialized treatments present a significant barrier to the widespread adoption of personalized healthcare. While these advanced technologies offer the promise of better and more tailored care, their financial burden often puts them out of reach for many patients and healthcare systems. This financial obstacle not only limits individual access to potentially life-changing treatments but also hampers the broader implementation of personalized healthcare paradigms, thereby perpetuating a cycle of inequality in medical care.

Resources

The requirement for state-of-the-art medical facilities and highly trained healthcare personnel adds another layer of complexity to the already challenging landscape of personalized healthcare. In affluent settings, these resources are often readily available, making it easier to implement customized treatment plans that could significantly improve patient outcomes. However, in less wealthy regions or healthcare systems with fewer resources, these conditions can severely limit the feasibility of delivering personalized care. This stark contrast exacerbates healthcare disparities, denying those in less privileged settings the benefits of tailored treatments and diagnostics. As a result, the gap widens between what is medically possible and what is practically accessible, particularly in under-resourced communities.

Lack of Evidence

The absence of robust, long-term evidence to substantiate the effectiveness of personalized healthcare poses a considerable barrier to its widespread adoption. Many healthcare providers remain cautious, if not skeptical, about fully embracing customized treatments, often citing the dearth of large-scale, peer-reviewed studies as a reason for their hesitance.

This uncertainty can stifle innovation and hinder the incorporation of potentially transformative personalized healthcare solutions into mainstream medical practice. It creates a catch-22 situation: Without ample evidence, providers are reluctant to proceed, but that evidence can only be garnered through broader implementation and rigorous study of these personalized approaches. Consequently, this gap in empirical support not only slows down the evolution of healthcare but can also mean missed opportunities for improved patient outcomes.

Private sector funding and support require some justification of the practical reality of these treatment methodologies. The corporations that can play a significant role in helping realize the personalized healthcare agenda are not the type to gamble. Real-world data with expected return on investment, as well as validation that personalization will actually have a significant impact on patient wellness on a large scale, are required. Additionally, viability studies evaluating personalized healthcare for everyone will need to be completed.

Ethical Concerns

The reliance of personalized healthcare on an extensive array of patient data—from genetic profiles to lifestyle choices—brings into sharp focus ethical issues surrounding patient privacy and data security. As healthcare systems aggregate and analyze more individualized data to fine-tune treatment plans, they risk exposing sensitive information to potential misuse or unauthorized access.

These concerns are not merely hypothetical; they represent a palpable tension between the push for customized care and the obligation to safeguard patient confidentiality. These complex ethical issues will have to be addressed by healthcare organizations, balancing the revolutionary promise of data-driven individualized treatment against the imperative to maintain the privacy and trust of their patients. Ensuring robust cybersecurity measures and ethical protocols are in place is critical, as any breach in data security could have far-reaching implications, not only legally but also in terms of eroding patient trust in the healthcare system at large.

Ethical Disclosure

A dilemma arises when extensive portions of a patient's genome are sequenced and analyzed. Physicians are bound by the principle of Ethical Disclosure, which mandates that they share all medical findings with the patient. Yet, in certain cases, specific genetic data might indicate a predisposition towards severe, untreatable diseases. Once this predisposition is identified, it must be communicated to the patient. The ethical quandary emerges from the potential negative mental health effects of disclosing such information, particularly when there's no guarantee that the disease will ever develop. Is it justifiable to induce significant anxiety in a patient over a potential condition that might never materialize? Obviously, healthcare has work to do in defining the dilemmas, outlining procedures for addressing potentially life-threatening conditions, and ensuring counselors are involved in the process.

Unrealistic Expectations

The advent of personalized healthcare carries with it the potential for inflated or misguided expectations about treatment outcomes among patients. While the promise of tailored treatments can offer newfound hope, it can also cultivate a perception that personalized medicine is a guaranteed fix for complex health issues. When these heightened expectations aren't met, the result is often dissatisfaction and erosion of trust in healthcare providers and the system as a whole.

This sense of disillusionment can have a cascading effect, affecting patient compliance with ongoing treatments and willingness to engage in future healthcare initiatives. For healthcare providers, managing these expectations becomes a delicate balancing act—educating patients on the realistic outcomes of personalized healthcare without dampening their optimism for what could indeed be life-altering medical interventions. This makes effective communication and patient education crucial components in the successful implementation of personalized healthcare models.

Other Contributing Factors

There has been a major increase in the world population in the last 100 years, and yet there has not been an equal increase in hospital capacity to mirror it. An example that typifies this trend is Canada. According to the Canadian Museum of History (2010), in 1929, there were approximately 954 fully functional public and private hospitals operational in the country while its population from a census in 1926 was approximately 9,451,000 people. According to Statista.com (2016), there are now 1,300 hospitals in Canada while the population is 38.21 million. This represents a 36.3% increase in the number of hospitals, and yet there has been a 304.5%

growth in population. This statistical trend has occurred in most countries around the world and is the main contributor to the immense strain and overtaxing of healthcare industry resources, stretched thin due to insufficient capacity and understaffing.

It is expected that understaffing in the industry will only get worse. In recent years, it has been documented that the public interest in attending college overall has declined. According to Chambers (2019), of the World Economic Forum, the interest children have is not at all related to the jobs of the future. More and more, the rhetoric among the youth is that they desire to be entertainers or self-employed entrepreneurs. "Hustle" and "Grindset" cultures have made people desire to be their own boss and set their own hours. A society cannot survive with entertainers and entrepreneurs alone. Basic public service and infrastructure development/ maintenance jobs are no longer desired.

AI for Enhanced Patient Outcomes

The Role of AI in Personalizing Treatment Plans

The true strength of artificial intelligence in healthcare manifests in its unparalleled capacity for data analysis— analyzing intricate, large-scale data sets at a speed and accuracy that far surpass human capabilities. For physicians, this means having an advanced analytical tool at their disposal that can swiftly sift through layers of medical records, genetic information, and even real-time biometric data. By doing so, AI provides deep, actionable insights that can be invaluable in formulating treatment plans tailored specifically to each patient's unique medical profile. Rather than relying on generalized treatment protocols or time-consuming trial-and-error methods, physicians can leverage AI's predictive analytics to identify which treatments are most likely to be effective for individual patients.

This not only enhances the quality of care but also reduces the chances of adverse side effects and failed treatments, thereby conserving both time and medical resources. Overall, AI serves as an indispensable partner in the healthcare provider's quest to deliver more personalized and effective patient care.

AI Solutions to the Challenges of Personalized Healthcare

Artificial intelligence possesses remarkable capabilities that can significantly alleviate various obstacles commonly associated with the delivery of personalized healthcare. One of the most immediate benefits is AI's ability to automate routine tasks—such as data collection and analysis—that traditionally require significant human labor. This automation not only streamlines operational workflows but also has the potential to drive down the costs associated with these activities. By doing so, AI makes personalized healthcare approaches more financially accessible to a wider patient base.

Additionally, AI can optimize the utilization of medical resources through intelligent scheduling, patient triage, and resource allocation, ensuring that the right patients receive the right care at the right time. This leads to more efficient use of existing resources, which is particularly beneficial in settings that may not have abundant resources to begin with.

Maintaining patient privacy is a paramount concern. AI offers advanced encryption and anonymization techniques that can secure patient data while still making it usable for medical research and treatment planning.

Patient-Centric Cure Development and Medicinal Research

The Digital Revolution in Clinical Research

The healthcare landscape is undergoing a transformation, largely fueled by advancements in artificial intelligence and digital technology. These technologies are not merely add-ons; they are integral components shaping a new paradigm where collaboration between clinical researchers and patients takes center stage.

This increasing collaboration is more than just a trend—it's a catalyst that is enhancing the quality of medical research in significant ways. By facilitating a more interactive and participatory research process it directly influences critical aspects like safety standards and the effectiveness of drug therapies. In other words, the synergy between AI, digital technology, and a more collaborative healthcare environment is setting the stage for a future where medicine is not only more advanced but also more attuned to the individual needs of patients.

Tailored Preventive and Therapeutic Interventions

With the unprecedented availability of comprehensive patient data, clinicians are now equipped with information that ranges from genetic makeup to lifestyle factors. This data is not just informational; it's transformational. It provides healthcare professionals with the unique capability to design highly targeted and specific medical interventions tailored to individual patient needs.

"On a broader level, by reducing avoidable unnecessary outpatient and inpatient events, stakeholders can relieve the overall health system capacity" (Bestsennyy & Cordina, 2021). Up to 30% of readmissions are considered avoidable if better post-discharge patient care is given.

The result is a dual benefit: a measurable improvement in patient outcomes and a potential reduction in healthcare costs. By identifying more effective treatments the first time around, healthcare systems can avoid the often-exorbitant expenses associated with trial-and-error approaches, thus streamlining care and enhancing patient satisfaction.

Cost and Convenience

The capability of AI to accurately identify the most suitable treatments goes beyond mere clinical effectiveness; it has substantial economic and logistical benefits as well. By using AI algorithms to sift through a myriad of possible interventions and highlight those most likely to succeed for a specific patient, healthcare providers can substantially cut costs associated with less effective or redundant treatments.

This not only minimizes the financial burden on both the healthcare system and patients but also reduces the inconvenience associated with prolonged or ineffective treatment regimens. In essence, AI serves as a powerful tool in streamlining the healthcare process, making it not just more personalized but also more efficient and cost-effective.

In America, sequencing the first genome took many decades, billions of dollars in investments (approximately $3.8 billion), and contributions from the entire scientific community. Today, it is nearing $100, and it is possible to fully map the entire genome within 24 hours, even with the slower working speed of humans and somewhat dated computer technology in most hospitals (Office of Science, 2015; Jennings, 2020).

Conclusion

The synergy between AI technology and the objective of personalized healthcare stands as a groundbreaking shift towards a new era of individualized, precise, and effective medical treatment. This alignment has the power to overcome existing challenges, transforming the way healthcare is delivered and experienced. However, it's worth noting that some critics argue that the priority should be on achieving universal healthcare coverage before venturing into AI-driven personalized medicine. They contend that before we invest in optimizing healthcare for everyone, it is crucial to ensure that basic healthcare services are accessible to all. Despite these concerns, proponents of AI in healthcare argue that the technology not only makes treatment more effective but also more efficient, potentially making healthcare more accessible in the long term. Indeed, the marriage of AI and personalized healthcare brings with it the tantalizing promise of a future where healthcare is not just universally accessible, but also uniquely tailored to everyone's needs.

Chapter 6:

AI in Healthcare: Limitations

Safeguarding the Future of AI in Healthcare: Ethical and Practical Considerations

The power and sophistication of AI are increasing at a dizzying rate. Consider the following example of just how potent these systems can be. In a recent study, a team from NYU's Tandon School of Engineering crafted virtual fingerprints that deceived fingerprint readers in 22% of instances (NYU Tandon School of Engineering, 2018). This unsettling finding implies that nearly one in four devices relying on such biometric authentication could potentially be compromised. As AI becomes more integrated into healthcare, the stakes for safeguarding against such vulnerabilities rise exponentially.

"Fingerprint-based authentication is still a strong way to protect a device or a system, but at this point, most systems don't verify whether a fingerprint or other biometric is coming from a real person or a replica," said Bontrager. "These experiments demonstrate the need for multi-factor authentication and should be a wake-up call for device manufacturers about the potential for artificial fingerprint attacks" (NYU Tandon School of Engineering, 2018).

Ethical Considerations of AI in Healthcare

Safeguarding Patient Data

The undeniable transformative power of artificial intelligence in healthcare paves the way for innovations ranging from diagnostics to individualized treatments. However, this revolutionary shift comes with its own set of risks, most notably patient data privacy. As AI algorithms require access to extensive databases of personal health records to operate effectively, the stakes for potential data breaches become alarmingly high. Even a single security lapse could expose a treasure trove of sensitive information, ranging from medical histories and test results to financial and demographic data.

Patients need to have the utmost confidence that their personal information is being handled with care and safeguarded to the highest standards. This requires not just strong encryption methods, but also a well-rounded framework encompassing data governance policies, access management, and routine security evaluations. Additionally, as AI healthcare applications often involve multiple stakeholders—including healthcare providers, software vendors, and potentially even third-party researchers—ensuring secure and ethical data-sharing practices becomes even more complex.

Aside from technical safeguards, there is also a growing need for clear, accessible communication about data privacy policies. Patients should be fully informed about how their data is being used, who has access to it, and what measures are in place to protect it. This is not just a matter of legal compliance; it's a crucial step in building and maintaining trust between healthcare providers and their patients, which is foundational for the successful adoption of AI in healthcare.

While AI holds the promise of drastically improving patient care, the risks it poses to patient data privacy are substantial and must be rigorously managed. Balancing the incredible potential of AI with the imperative to protect patient data presents one of the most critical challenges facing the healthcare industry today.

Patient Consent

The advent of AI in healthcare brings about a myriad of opportunities for better diagnosis, personalized treatment, and overall enhanced patient experience. However, the opaque nature of some AI algorithms—often described as a "black box" for their lack of interpretability—raises significant ethical concerns, especially in the realm of patient consent. In traditional medical settings, informed consent is a cornerstone of ethical practice, ensuring that patients understand the treatments they are receiving and the associated risks. The complexity and unpredictability of AI algorithms complicate this model of informed consent, as even experts sometimes struggle to interpret exactly how decisions are made.

Patients have the right not just to know that AI is being used in their healthcare but also to understand, to the extent possible, how it is being used. This entails a comprehensive explanation of what data the AI will analyze, what kinds of decisions it might make, and how those decisions could impact their treatment or diagnosis. While the technical details may be complex, healthcare providers have an ethical obligation to ensure that this information is presented in an understandable manner. This might mean using layman's terms, analogies, or other explanatory models to clarify the algorithm's function.

Moreover, the informed consent process should be continuous, not a one-time event. As AI algorithms are often updated or even learn from new data, it's crucial that patients are kept in the loop about changes that might impact their care. This could be particularly pertinent if the AI system will be used for ongoing monitoring or if the algorithm will be updated during treatment.

Another aspect to consider is the role of regulatory oversight to ensure that informed consent protocols are being consistently and rigorously upheld. This could include third-party audits, as well as the potential for patients to revoke their consent if they are uncomfortable with how their data is being used.

The increasing role of AI in healthcare necessitates a reevaluation and strengthening of existing informed consent protocols. This is critical not just for ethical compliance but also for building and maintaining the trust that is fundamental to the healthcare provider-patient relationship.

Addressing Patient Bias

The use of AI in healthcare holds enormous potential for improving diagnosis and treatment outcomes, but its effectiveness is closely tied to the quality and diversity of the data sets used in training the algorithms. When AI models are trained on biased, skewed, or incomplete data, they risk not only making inaccurate predictions but also perpetuating existing disparities in healthcare. For instance, if an algorithm designed to identify skin cancer is primarily trained on data from lighter-skinned individuals, its ability to accurately diagnose darker-skinned people could be compromised, leading to delayed or incorrect treatment.

The issue of bias isn't limited to ethnic or racial disparities; it can also manifest in terms of age, gender, socioeconomic status, and other factors that can influence health outcomes. This is particularly problematic as healthcare strives for equity, providing all individuals, regardless of their background, with the best possible standard of care. Consequently, rigorous safeguards and continuous monitoring need to be implemented to ensure that AI algorithms are as unbiased as possible.

Addressing this challenge can be approached by utilizing training data that is diverse and representative. This involves gathering comprehensive data that accurately reflects the variety of patients the AI tool is likely to encounter. Another strategy is to incorporate *fairness algorithms* that can identify and correct biases in the data. Furthermore, it's crucial that any AI model used in healthcare undergoes stringent validation procedures, including testing its performance across diverse demographic groups. These steps can help ensure that AI tools contribute to reducing systemic inequalities rather than exacerbating them.

In addition, transparency about the limitations of AI models is essential. Clinicians, healthcare administrators, and patients should be aware of any biases or limitations inherent in AI tools being used. Ongoing audits and impact assessments can provide valuable insights into the real-world implications of AI algorithms, offering an opportunity to make necessary adjustments.

Ultimately, the goal is to create AI tools that are not only technically proficient but also ethically sound, facilitating equitable healthcare outcomes for all patient populations.

Scenarios to Consider

The Complexity of Accountability in Faulty AI Diagnosis

Picture a medical setting where an advanced AI diagnostic system is used as an integral part of healthcare delivery. A patient, Jane, visits her healthcare provider concerned about a set of symptoms she has been experiencing that could be indicative of a severe condition like cancer. The provider uses an AI diagnostic tool to analyze Jane's symptoms, medical history, and preliminary test results. The AI system, which has been statistically reliable in the past, concludes that Jane does not have cancer and suggests that her symptoms are likely due to a less severe condition. Relying on this diagnosis, Jane decides to forgo further testing and treatment, such as biopsies or imaging scans, that would otherwise have been the next steps in a traditional diagnostic process.

Months later, Jane's condition worsens dramatically. A second opinion and additional tests reveal that she does, in fact, have advanced cancer that has now progressed to a stage where treatment options are limited and less effective. Tragically, the delayed diagnosis has severe consequences for Jane's health and quality of life.

This scenario raises a complex web of ethical and legal questions. Who bears the responsibility for the faulty diagnosis? Is it the healthcare provider who placed trust in the AI system? Is it the developers or operators of the AI diagnostic tool that provided an incorrect analysis? Or does some level of accountability fall on Jane for choosing to rely on a single diagnostic avenue?

In cases like this, the issue of liability becomes increasingly complicated. Traditional medical malpractice frameworks may not be fully equipped to handle errors made by a machine, especially when human healthcare providers also have some level of trust and reliance on the technology. The lines between human error and technological failure blur, creating a legal and ethical gray area that the healthcare industry and legal systems are still navigating.

Furthermore, scenarios like this highlight the critical need for checks and balances in AI healthcare applications. It points to the importance of human oversight and the necessity of multiple layers of diagnostic verification, especially in life-or-death cases such as cancer diagnosis. It also calls attention to the importance of fully informing patients about the role of AI in their healthcare and the limitations that these systems might have, thus giving patients the information they need to make informed decisions.

This scenario underscores the urgent need for clear guidelines and regulations concerning AI in healthcare, not only to assign accountability but also to prevent such tragic outcomes from happening in the first place.

The Aftermath of a Data Breach in AI-Driven Healthcare Systems

Picture a state-of-the-art hospital that employs cutting-edge AI technologies for various purposes, ranging from predictive analytics for patient outcomes to intelligent electronic health record management. Despite robust security measures, a sophisticated cyber-attacker identifies and exploits a vulnerability in the AI system, gaining unauthorized access to an extensive database containing thousands of confidential patient records, treatment plans, medications, and medical histories.

Upon discovery of the breach, the hospital's immediate response is to secure the compromised system to prevent further data leakage. The IT department works around the clock to identify the exploited vulnerability and patch it, but the damage is done. The compromised data is extensive, affecting not just the patients but also the trust placed in the institution and, by extension, the acceptability of AI technologies in healthcare.

- **Legal Obligations:** In compliance with privacy laws such as the Health Insurance Portability and

Accountability Act (HIPAA) in the United States, the hospital is legally required to inform affected patients of the breach. Failure to do so in a timely manner could result in severe fines and legal action.

- **Restoring Trust:** The hospital initiates a multi-pronged strategy to regain public trust. This involves transparent communication about the breach, what steps are being taken to prevent future occurrences, and offering affected patients free identity protection services. Crisis communication experts are consulted to guide public announcements and patient notifications.

- **Technical Safeguards:** On the technical side, the hospital conducts a thorough audit of its AI and cybersecurity systems to identify potential weaknesses. Additional layers of security are implemented, such as two-factor authentication, advanced encryption methods, and frequent, randomized security audits.

- **Revisiting Protocols:** The incident serves as a catalyst for the hospital to review and revise its data security protocols. Staff undergo renewed training on data protection, emphasizing the critical role each individual plays in maintaining data integrity.

- **Community and Patient Engagement:** A series of community engagement activities, like workshops and seminars on data privacy, are conducted to educate the public and patients on how they can protect their data and what steps the hospital has taken to safeguard their information.

- **Regulatory Review:** The incident may lead to a broader review of regulations governing the use of AI in healthcare, including a re-evaluation of existing compliance and monitoring mechanisms to ensure they are robust enough to prevent future breaches.

This unfortunate scenario serves as a stark reminder that while AI can offer remarkable benefits in healthcare, it also presents new avenues for vulnerabilities that can have severe repercussions on patient safety and trust. It highlights the continuous need for robust, adaptive cybersecurity measures and crisis management strategies to mitigate the impact of breaches when they do occur.

Addressing Discriminatory Outcomes Arising from Biased Algorithms

In this hypothetical scenario, a state-of-the-art hospital employs an advanced machine-learning algorithm to assess the necessity and urgency of surgeries. The goal is to optimize resource allocation, ensuring that surgeries are performed on those who need them most urgently. However, it soon becomes apparent that the algorithm disproportionately denies necessary surgeries to members of a marginalized community, essentially perpetuating and institutionalizing systemic discrimination within the healthcare system.

- **Immediate Remedial Actions:** As soon as this disparity is discovered, the use of the algorithm is suspended for review. An interdisciplinary team composed of data scientists, medical professionals, ethicists, and representatives from affected communities is assembled to scrutinize the algorithm.

- **Identifying the Source of Bias:** The team explores the algorithm's training data and methodology to identify the source of bias. This could range from the underrepresentation of certain groups in the training data to the algorithm learning from historical decisions made by healthcare providers, which could also be biased.

- **Algorithm Correction:** Once the source of the bias is identified, efforts are made to correct it. This could involve balancing the training dataset with more diverse data or tweaking the algorithm to counteract known biases. The revised algorithm is then tested rigorously to ensure that it does not produce discriminatory outcomes.

- **Validation and Auditing:** Independent third parties may be called upon to validate that the algorithm no longer produces biased results. Ongoing audits could be implemented to ensure the algorithm stays unbiased as it continues to learn from new data.

- **Legal and Ethical Considerations:** The hospital might need to deal with legal challenges from those who were unfairly denied surgeries. Ethical considerations must also be addressed, involving an open dialogue with the affected community to acknowledge the problem, describe the steps taken to correct it, and provide assurances for the future.

- **Transparency and Community Engagement:** Transparency in both the problem and the solution is key to rebuilding trust. The hospital can engage with the community through forums, seminars, or public consultations to discuss what went wrong and what steps have been taken to rectify the situation. Public input could also be sought in shaping policies or procedures that concern the use of AI in healthcare.

- **Institutional Changes:** The incident serves as an awakening for not just the hospital but the broader healthcare community about the hidden dangers of AI biases. It leads to the creation of guidelines or best practices for the use of AI in healthcare decision-making, emphasizing the need for ongoing monitoring for any form of discrimination.

By treating this alarming incident as both a learning opportunity and a call for systemic change, the hospital and healthcare community at large can take essential steps to ensure that AI is used in a way that is not just efficient but also equitable. This could serve as a vital lesson for the development and deployment of AI in healthcare, highlighting the necessity of continuous ethical scrutiny.

AI has enormous potential to benefit the healthcare sector, but only if integrated thoughtfully and securely. Ethical considerations like patient data privacy, consent, bias, and accountability cannot be afterthoughts; they must be integral components of any AI healthcare strategy. Strict guidelines, limitations, and safety measures need to be established to harness the power of AI responsibly, thus ensuring a future where AI aids healthcare without compromising integrity and trust.

Chapter 6:

Part 2:
AI Ethics and Regulations

Patient Consent: The Ethical Bedrock of AI in Healthcare

The Time-Honored Importance of Consent in Medicine

Patient consent is not merely a formality; it is an ethical and legal obligation that ensures respect for individual autonomy and human dignity. From routine tests to major surgeries, physicians have long made it a point to obtain informed consent from patients or their legally authorized representatives. This practice embodies a social contract that places trust and understanding between healthcare providers and those they serve. In essence, it represents a shared decision-making process that honors the patient's perspective and empowers them to make informed choices about their care.

The Complexities of Consent in the Age of AI

In the world of AI-driven healthcare, the concept of informed consent becomes more complex. Here, the decision-making process involves more than just the interaction between the physician and the patient. It extends to machine algorithms that operate under a set of rules not easily understood even by experts. Consequently, the *informed* part of *informed consent* faces new challenges. Can patients be said to have granted their consent if they don't fully understand the algorithms that may determine their treatment?

Transparency and Explainability

One way to address this is by enhancing the transparency and explainability of AI algorithms. Patients should be provided with easily understandable information about how AI will be involved in their diagnosis or treatment. While the technicalities of machine learning models might be difficult to convey, the aim should be to demystify the technology enough for patients to make genuinely informed decisions.

Continuous Consent

Traditional consent is often a one-time event, but with AI's ability to continuously analyze data and adapt recommendations, the concept of *continuous consent* may need to be introduced. This involves regularly updating the patient on any changes in AI-driven treatment plans and seeking their ongoing approval.

Digital Consent Forms and AI Summaries

Modernizing the informed consent process could include digital consent forms that can be updated in real time. These digital forms might also feature AI-generated summaries explaining the rationale behind diagnostics or treatments. This information should be conveyed in a manner that is understandable to laypersons, ensuring that they are actively involved in the decision-making process.

The Importance of Ethical Guidelines and Regulatory Oversight

Considering the multifaceted ethical and practical complexities surrounding the application of AI in healthcare, there's an urgent need for comprehensive ethical guidelines and regulatory oversight. These guidelines should be formulated through interdisciplinary collaboration involving medical professionals, data scientists, ethicists, and legal experts to ensure a holistic approach. They must explicitly detail the criteria and procedures for obtaining informed consent from patients when their data will be analyzed by AI algorithms, ensuring that individuals are fully aware of how their information will be used and what implications it might have for their treatment.

Transparency should be a cornerstone of these guidelines. Patients must have the right to know not just that AI is being used but also how it's being used, including the types of algorithms in play and the data sources being analyzed. Transparency extends to healthcare providers as well; there should be clarity about the decision-making process, and patients should be provided the opportunity to contest decisions made predominantly or exclusively by AI.

Data privacy also needs meticulous attention in these guidelines. With AI capable of analyzing vast and sensitive sets of personal health records, stringent measures must be in place to safeguard this data. This includes advanced encryption methods, regular security audits, and quick response mechanisms to address any security breaches.

Accountability forms another crucial component of these regulations. In case of errors or issues such as misdiagnosis or data breaches, it must be clearly outlined who bears the responsibility and what corrective actions will be taken. This not only helps in mitigating the risks but also aids in re-establishing patient trust.

Moreover, these guidelines should be dynamic and open to regular updates, as AI technology and its applications in healthcare are continuously evolving. Public and patient input should be considered in these updates to ensure that the regulations remain aligned with societal values and expectations.

By implementing robust ethical guidelines and regulatory oversight, we can manage the complex landscape of AI in healthcare more safely and effectively, optimizing its immense potential while minimizing risks.

The Evolution of Informed Consent: Maintaining Core Ethical Principles

As artificial intelligence technologies become increasingly implemented into healthcare, it's imperative that our strategies for ensuring informed consent adapt to keep pace. This doesn't mean, however, that the underlying ethical bedrock should waver. On the contrary, the fundamental principle—respecting and safeguarding the autonomy and dignity of each patient—should remain immutable and stand as a guiding light for navigating the challenges that AI brings to healthcare decision-making.

While AI offers remarkable advantages in diagnosing and treating illnesses, its complexity and "black box" nature often make it difficult for patients to fully understand the implications of consenting to its use. In this scenario, our methodology towards informed consent necessitates a contemporary reevaluation. The patient must be made aware not just of the benefits and risks of the traditional treatment pathways but also of the specific consequences, uncertainties, and ethical considerations of involving AI in their care.

Furthermore, AI should not be seen as an entity separate from the healthcare system but as an integral part of it designed to serve the patient. As such, its introduction should serve to elevate, rather than erode, the time-honored ethical commitment to patient autonomy and informed consent. The dynamic nature of AI technologies, which are constantly evolving and improving, should act as a stimulus for healthcare providers to continually reassess and strengthen informed consent protocols. These protocols should be transparent, easily accessible, and inclusive, ensuring that patients from all backgrounds are equipped to make truly informed decisions about their healthcare.

In essence, while the introduction of AI into healthcare complicates the ethical and practical facets of informed consent, it also offers an opportunity to revisit and reinforce this critical principle, adapting it for an age of unprecedented medical complexity. This challenge and opportunity makes it clear that respecting patient autonomy and dignity is not merely a static requirement but a dynamic commitment that must evolve alongside technological advances.

The Complexity of Accountability in the Age of AI-Driven Healthcare

Accountability has long served as a cornerstone in the healthcare industry, providing a framework for ethical and effective practice. Traditionally, responsibility and liability have been clearly mapped out, usually resting on the shoulders of physicians, nurses, and healthcare institutions. These professionals and organizations are bound by an established set of rules and ethical guidelines, ensuring a degree of transparency and culpability in their actions.

However, the advent of AI-driven healthcare has introduced an unprecedented level of complexity to this equation. When an AI system makes an incorrect recommendation, or otherwise fails to perform as expected, the ripple effects extend far beyond the patient-provider relationship. Suddenly, we're thrust into a complex network involving software developers who built the AI, healthcare providers who implemented it, and regulatory bodies that approved its use. The traditional lines of accountability become blurred, making it difficult to pinpoint who exactly should be held responsible when things go awry.

Is the liability on the developers who may have failed to account for certain variables or biases in their algorithms? Or should healthcare providers bear the brunt for relying too heavily on a still-evolving technology? And what role do regulatory agencies play in this puzzle, especially if they were the ones to approve the AI system for medical use in the first place?

This calls for a reevaluation of existing accountability frameworks. New models of responsibility must be developed to encompass the multifaceted interactions between human healthcare providers and artificial intelligence systems. These models should clarify how liability is determined and shared among the various parties involved, thereby ensuring that patients have clear paths to recourse and that responsible parties are appropriately held to account. In an age where AI has the potential to both greatly enhance and complicate healthcare delivery, revisiting and updating our understanding of accountability is not just beneficial—it's imperative.

*The Role of Developers and Engineers in the
Accountability Ecosystem*

In the context of AI in healthcare, the responsibility of developers and engineers extends well beyond the act of creating the software. They are tasked with ensuring that the algorithms are not just functional but also accurate, reliable, and free from biases that could compromise patient care. They must rigorously validate these systems, applying rigorous scientific methods to ensure the algorithms perform as intended across a wide range of scenarios and patient demographics.

Moreover, the responsibility doesn't end after the software is deployed. Developers are obligated to continually monitor their AI systems for both performance and ethical considerations, identifying vulnerabilities or potential areas for misuse. Security is another significant concern; developers must release updates and patches to address any security risks that could expose sensitive patient information or otherwise harm individuals.

In cases where an AI system has led to an error or harmful outcome, the burden falls on the developers to meticulously investigate the issue. They must determine whether the fault lies in the algorithm itself, the data it was trained on, or the manner in which it was implemented in the healthcare setting. Once identified, immediate steps must be taken to rectify the issue, whether through software updates, retraining the algorithm, or issuing guidelines for its more appropriate use.

The stakes are incredibly high. Any lapse in these areas not only risks harm to patients but also threatens the broader adoption of AI technologies in healthcare. Therefore, the role of developers and engineers in this ecosystem is pivotal and requires an ongoing commitment to ethical development, transparency, and collaboration with other stakeholders in healthcare.

The Multifaceted Responsibilities of Healthcare Providers

Healthcare providers carry a substantial burden of responsibility when it comes to incorporating AI technologies into their practice. While these systems offer promising advancements in diagnostics, treatment planning, and even patient management, medical professionals are still the final arbiters of patient care. This makes it imperative for them to fully understand both the capabilities and limitations of the AI tools they are using.

Their role is not just operational but also educational. Healthcare providers must keep themselves up to date with the latest advancements and updates in AI technologies relevant to their field. This involves not only learning how to operate new systems but also comprehending the scientific principles that underlie these tools. They must be familiar with the type of data the AI uses, how it processes this data, and the reliability of its outputs under various conditions.

Moreover, their responsibility extends to ethical considerations. While AI can assist in decision-making, the ultimate responsibility for any treatment or diagnosis rests with the healthcare provider. This means they cannot abdicate their professional judgment solely to an algorithm, especially in complex or life-threatening cases. Ideally, AI serves as an additional tool for informed decision-making, supplementing but not replacing the healthcare provider's expertise.

Healthcare providers also have a responsibility to communicate openly with patients regarding how AI is utilized in their care process. This involves explaining what the technology can and cannot do and how it influences, but does not dictate, the overall treatment plan. Patients must feel confident that the human element—the expertise, experience, and ethical reasoning of their healthcare provider—remains central in their care, even in an environment increasingly influenced by AI.

Healthcare providers have a multifaceted role that spans understanding technology, continuous education, ethical decision-making, and transparent communication. Each of these aspects contributes to their shared accountability in the successful and ethical deployment of AI in healthcare.

The Expansive Role of Regulatory Agencies

Regulatory agencies, whether governmental or independent, play an absolutely critical role in the burgeoning field of AI in healthcare. These bodies bear the responsibility for not only ensuring that AI systems meet established safety and efficacy standards but also for monitoring their ongoing performance and ethical implications.

Firstly, these agencies are tasked with defining the criteria under which an AI system can be approved for use in healthcare settings. This typically involves a rigorous evaluation of the system's accuracy, reliability, and impact on patient outcomes. It may also extend to assessing the ethical dimensions, like ensuring that the AI does not reinforce existing healthcare disparities or violate privacy norms.

Once an AI system is in use, the role of the regulatory agency shifts to one of continuous monitoring and assessment. This means keeping track of any incidents where the AI system may have failed, misdiagnosed, or led to undesirable outcomes. They may also conduct or sponsor post-market studies to ensure that the AI tools are performing as expected and to identify any long-term risks or benefits that were not apparent during initial testing.

In cases where an AI system proves to be problematic—whether due to inaccuracy, ethical concerns, or other issues—

regulatory agencies have the authority to intervene. This could mean mandating updates or modifications to the system or, in extreme cases, calling for its temporary or permanent removal from the healthcare setting.

Additionally, regulatory agencies have a responsibility to the public to communicate clearly and transparently about the status of AI in healthcare. This might involve publishing guidelines for healthcare providers on how to use AI ethically and effectively or issuing public advisories in the event of significant problems with an AI system.

Lastly, these agencies often act as intermediaries between technology developers, healthcare providers, and the public. They may facilitate discussions or negotiations among these stakeholders to ensure that AI technologies are being deployed in a manner that is ethical, effective, and aligned with the public interest.

The role of regulatory agencies in AI-driven healthcare is comprehensive, spanning from initial approval to ongoing oversight, and involves a multiplicity of tasks aimed at safeguarding both individual and public health.

Worst-Case Scenarios: A Comprehensive, Three-Pronged Approach

1. Immediate Suspension: The First Line of Defense

In the event of a significant failure or harmful outcome stemming from the use of an AI system in healthcare, the immediate priority should be patient safety. The healthcare institution employing the AI system must promptly suspend its operation pending a thorough investigation. This action serves as a necessary, preemptive step to prevent further errors or harm. To ensure unbiased examination, the institution should consult with regulatory agencies, external experts, and potentially even the public to decide whether it's safe and appropriate to reinstate the system or if permanent discontinuation is warranted.

2. Preventive Measures: Root Cause Analysis and Rectification

Once the AI system is safely suspended, the next step is to identify the root cause of the failure. Both the AI developers and regulatory bodies should collaboratively dissect the issue, drawing from available data, logs, and expert opinion. Preventive actions can then be formulated based on these insights. These may range from simple software patches to more extensive overhauls, like reprogramming the algorithm or retraining it with a more diverse and robust data set. Preventive measures should also extend to updating guidelines and best practices for healthcare providers who interact with the AI system to ensure that similar mishaps are avoided in the future.

3. Reparative Actions: Legal and Ethical Accountability

After taking preventive measures, the focus should shift to reparative actions to compensate those harmed by the AI system's failure. This is a complex area that involves both legal and ethical considerations. On the legal front, healthcare providers may find themselves facing malpractice lawsuits, and AI developers could be subject to product liability claims. Ethically, both parties must transparently communicate the failure and their corrective actions to affected patients and the broader public.

Furthermore, healthcare institutions may also face reputational damage and could be liable for failing to implement adequate safeguards or for negligence in the usage of a faulty AI system. Reparative actions may include financial compensation, public apologies, or other forms of restitution that restore trust and integrity in the healthcare system.

A Collective Responsibility

In the evolving landscape of AI-driven healthcare, accountability is a shared responsibility that demands a coordinated, multi-layered approach. Rather than isolating blame or responsibility to a single entity, the focus should be on creating a comprehensive framework that involves developers, healthcare providers, and regulatory agencies. This framework should specify the roles and duties of each party and provide a roadmap for legal accountability. The goal is to ensure that as AI technologies become increasingly integrated into healthcare, they do so in a manner that is safe, ethical, and transparent for all stakeholders involved.

The Challenge of Tracking in AI-Driven Healthcare

Tracking the decision-making process within AI applications poses a significant hurdle, especially when a negative outcome occurs. The question arises: Can the technology be sufficiently transparent to allow us to identify the root cause of a problem, thereby enabling its prevention in future cases? The importance of tracking goes beyond just troubleshooting; it's crucial for establishing accountability among developers, healthcare providers, and regulatory agencies. To achieve this, several layers of the AI system must be easily accessible for scrutiny. This involves not only a thorough analysis of the algorithm's real-time decision logs but also a close examination of the validation data used to test the system's performance. Moreover, scrutiny should extend to the initial training data, which can hold clues about inherent biases or inconsistencies that may have impacted the AI's decisions. By dissecting these different elements, healthcare institutions can gain a detailed understanding of how and why an AI application arrived at a particular decision, which is critical for both immediate remediation and long-term improvements.

Mandatory Human Intervention: Drawing the Line in AI-Driven Healthcare

The promise of AI in transforming healthcare is undeniable, offering groundbreaking advancements in areas ranging from diagnostics to treatment optimization. However, the technology should not be viewed as a complete replacement for human skills, judgment, and emotional intelligence. In this rapidly evolving landscape, it becomes vital to explicitly define where AI can augment human capabilities and where human intervention is irreplaceable.

This is not merely a theoretical consideration; it has practical implications for patient safety, ethical considerations, and even legal accountability. Whether it's making a diagnosis that considers the patient's emotional and psychological state or navigating ethical dilemmas, there are domains in healthcare that still require the unique abilities that only humans possess. As we increasingly integrate AI into healthcare systems, creating a balanced framework that distinguishes between the responsibilities of AI and those of healthcare providers becomes not just desirable but essential for effective and ethical care.

The "Never-Delegate" List: Roles Reserved for Humans

- **Empathy and Emotional Support.** Healthcare is as much about treating the soul as it is about treating the body. Emotional well-being often affects physical health, and here, the human touch is irreplaceable. Physicians, nurses, and other healthcare providers offer empathy, active listening, and emotional support that are crucial for patient healing and comfort. While AI systems can manage data and analytics, they lack the emotional intelligence to sense the subtleties of human emotion and respond with genuine care.

- **Ethical Decision-Making.** Healthcare often involves managing complex ethical dilemmas—whether it's end-of-life care, resource allocation, or medical triage. Human clinicians bring to the table not only medical expertise but also a complex understanding of ethics, cultural sensitivities, and emotional factors. AI, with its current inability to fully comprehend these dimensions, should not be making these ethical decisions.

- **Complex Diagnostics.** AI has demonstrated prowess in analyzing large data sets, even identifying patterns that might be missed by human eyes. However, diagnosing a patient often involves piecing together information that is both quantitative and qualitative— like a patient's history, demeanor, or subjective experiences. The "art of diagnosis" lies in this synthesis, which remains a uniquely human skill.

- **Surgical Procedures.** Robotic surgeries, aided by AI, have shown promise in executing highly precise operations. However, these technologies are not yet capable of responding to the unexpected developments that can occur during surgery. Human expertise, intuition, and the ability to make real-time decisions based on tactile and visual cues remain essential in the surgical theater.

The Gray Areas: Shared Responsibilities

- **Continuous Monitoring.** AI can offer around-the-clock monitoring of patient vitals and can alert staff when parameters go out of range. But when an alarm goes off, it's the clinician who must decide the significance of that alarm. Is it a device malfunction, a temporary spike, or a real medical emergency? Human oversight is crucial for interpreting these anomalies.

- **Treatment Planning.** AI systems can sift through vast amounts of medical literature to propose evidence-based treatment options. However, the decision-making process doesn't stop at selecting a scientifically effective treatment. Clinicians must consider various other factors, such as the patient's lifestyle, potential side effects, coexisting conditions, and even the patient's wishes and beliefs. These elements demand human judgment in conjunction with AI recommendations.

Guidelines for Human-AI Collaboration in Healthcare

As we move closer to a future where AI plays an increasingly significant role in healthcare, the necessity for well-defined guidelines for human-AI interaction becomes paramount. These regulatory frameworks need to address several key areas to ensure the safe and ethical deployment of AI in clinical settings.

Decision Oversight

AI may be an excellent tool for sifting through massive amounts of data quickly, offering diagnostic suggestions or treatment options based on established criteria. However, these are just that—suggestions. The final decision, whether it's prescribing a medication or opting for a surgical procedure, should reside with qualified medical professionals. Human clinicians bring years of education, experience, and contextual understanding to the table, elements that AI cannot replicate.

Review Mechanisms

Given the evolving nature of both medicine and technology, it's essential to have periodic reviews of the performance of AI systems. Human experts should conduct these audits, focusing not just on the accuracy of AI predictions but also on identifying any biases in data that could lead to unequal healthcare outcomes. This process is crucial for continually refining the AI algorithms and ensuring that they are both fair and accurate.

Human-AI Interaction Training

It's not enough to simply install an AI system and expect healthcare providers to integrate it seamlessly into their workflow. Training programs should be in place to educate medical staff on how to collaborate effectively with AI tools. These programs should cover the technical aspects, such as how to interpret AI-generated reports, as well as ethical considerations, like when human judgment should override AI recommendations.

Complementary, Not Supplementary: Defining the Human-AI Balance in Healthcare

Artificial intelligence is a formidable asset that can revolutionize healthcare, from data analytics to predictive diagnostics. However, it's crucial to remember that its role should be complementary to human expertise rather than serving as a substitute. There are specific realms within healthcare that are inherently human-centric and should remain so for several compelling reasons.

Firstly, the emotional and psychological dimensions of healthcare are elements that no AI can replicate. Whether it's the compassionate touch of a nurse or the reassuring words of a doctor, human interactions play a pivotal role in patient recovery and well-being. These aspects of care contribute to the holistic treatment of a patient, extending beyond mere medical interventions.

Secondly, the ethical landscape of healthcare often presents intimate dilemmas that require an intricate understanding of human values, cultural norms, and moral principles. These are areas where human judgment is indispensable because they involve not just factual considerations but a comprehensive understanding of human complexities.

Thirdly, while AI can sift through volumes of data to suggest a diagnosis or treatment, the final clinical decision often involves variables that can't be easily quantified, such as a patient's personal preferences, ethical beliefs, and long-term life goals. It's the human healthcare provider who synthesizes all these factors into a cohesive treatment plan.

Quality Control: An Ethical Imperative and Technical Necessity

In the race to integrate artificial intelligence into healthcare, we must not overlook the essential component of quality control. Machine learning algorithms, which form the core of most AI applications in healthcare, operate based on the data they're trained on and the programming logic that underpins them. Therefore, the accuracy and reliability of the data used for training these algorithms are not just technical requirements but ethical imperatives.

Firstly, the quality of data directly impacts the performance of the AI system. Poorly curated or imprecise data can lead to incorrect diagnoses, flawed treatment plans, and even severe health risks. Ensuring data quality means rigorous data validation processes, including cross-referencing with other credible sources and continual updating to include the most recent medical research.

"But even those who see AI's potential value recognize its potential risks. Poorly designed systems can misdiagnose. Software trained on data sets that reflect cultural biases will incorporate those blind spots" (Powell, 2020).

Secondly, data reliability is of utmost importance. Data used in healthcare AI systems should originate from reputable databases and should undergo multiple rounds of verification to rule out any inconsistencies. Inconsistent data can produce erratic behavior in AI systems, which, in healthcare settings, can have life-altering or even life-threatening consequences.

Recent studies have revealed that many published research findings are frequently inaccurate. Moreover, it has been observed that studies with false findings tend to garner more attention and citations, likely due to their surprising results (Huded et al, 2013). The reasons behind these inaccuracies can vary widely and are hard to pinpoint. However, primary causes include flawed testing parameters, issues with experimental procedures, unreliable data collection methods, and small or inconclusive sample sizes. Additionally, there have been recent instances where researchers intentionally manipulated results for personal benefit and to support their hypotheses (Ioannidis, 2005; Smith, 2021).

Thirdly, data accuracy is vital for building trust among healthcare providers and patients. Healthcare practitioners need to be assured that the AI tools they employ are dependable. Patients, in turn, need to have faith that the algorithms advising their healthcare providers are both safe and effective. A compromise in data accuracy can undermine this trust and slow down the adoption of what could be transformative healthcare technology.

The Foundational Importance of Data Quality

Training a machine learning model is an intricate process that hinges on the quality of data it's fed. Quality, in this context, encapsulates multiple dimensions: comprehensiveness, diversity, accuracy, and freedom from biases. Recognizing AI's transformative potential must go hand-in-hand with an awareness of its inherent limitations. When AI systems are built on poorly designed datasets, the outcomes could range from erroneous diagnoses to harmful treatment plans, effectively embedding existing cultural and social biases into healthcare decision-making.

That's a balancing act that industry stakeholders and developers have to execute flawlessly. The potential of this technology warrants that level of attention to detail and commitment. Successfully vetting and potentially reformatting data will significantly slow the process, yet it is crucial that it be executed correctly.

The High Stakes of Poor Data

The cost of training AI models on inadequate or biased data isn't just academic; it's a matter of life and death. Such scenarios could lead to misdiagnosis, incorrect treatment suggestions, and even severe physical harm. To mitigate this, data should undergo rigorous validation processes that verify its integrity, relevance, and applicability in real-world clinical settings.

One of the critical challenges in AI deployment is its tendency to perpetuate cultural or demographic biases found in the training data. This necessitates meticulous auditing and cleansing of the data to ensure that the AI system delivers equitable healthcare solutions across diverse patient populations.

A Multi-Stakeholder Approach to Quality Control

Effective quality control can't be the sole purview of any single group; it requires a collaborative effort involving data scientists, software developers, healthcare practitioners, and even regulatory agencies. This network of oversight should include specialized Data Validation Teams comprising domain experts to ensure clinical relevance. Additionally, third-party audits add another layer of scrutiny, eliminating blind spots that the primary team might overlook. Regulatory compliance ensures that AI systems meet the pre-established safety and efficacy criteria.

The Need for Real-Time Monitoring

Given the real-time demands of healthcare applications, quality control mechanisms must also function in real time. This entails immediate flagging of anomalies or unreliable data points that could otherwise skew the AI's decision-making processes, leading to suboptimal or even harmful outcomes.

A Continual Commitment to Excellence

Quality control in AI-driven healthcare is not merely a launch-phase requirement; it's an ongoing commitment. The repercussions of lapses are too grave to permit any level of complacency. By instituting a multi-layered, continually updated quality control framework, we do more than ensure the technical efficacy of AI in healthcare. We also fortify the ethical bulwarks that should be non-negotiable in medical practice.

By combining these elements together, we emphasize the foundational importance of data quality as both a technical necessity and an ethical imperative, ensuring the responsible and effective deployment of AI in healthcare.

We've explored the multifaceted ethical and practical considerations that come with integrating AI into healthcare. From the fundamental need for patient consent to the complex issues surrounding accountability, it's clear that unbridled AI has potential risks that must be managed carefully. The necessity for human intervention in specific healthcare roles underscores the irreplaceable value of human expertise and emotional intelligence. Lastly, stringent quality control measures are non-negotiable to ensure data reliability and, by extension, the safety and effectiveness of AI in healthcare. As we advance into this new frontier, imposing thoughtful limits and safeguards is not just prudent; it's a moral imperative.

Chapter 7:

AI Challenges

Despite AI's tremendous potential for positive change, its integration remains fraught with numerous challenges that are both practical and psychological. By outlining the specifics, I hope to clarify why AI in healthcare has not yet reached its full promise.

The Fallibility of Epic AI's Algorithms—A Cautionary Tale

One of the most glaring examples illustrating the potential fallibility of AI in healthcare is the case of Epic AI's algorithms. According to a 2021 STAT investigation, the system, designed to assist healthcare professionals by providing accurate and relevant information, fell far short of its promises.

The Context

Epic AI has created algorithms intended to transform healthcare information delivery, promising to offer actionable insights for better patient outcomes. The healthcare industry watched with great anticipation, envisioning a future where doctors could make quick, data-driven decisions, thereby saving lives and reducing costs.

The Reality: A Systemic Failure

Despite the hype and promise, the algorithms demonstrated significant shortcomings when put into practice. The system often failed to deliver relevant or accurate information, sometimes recommending treatments that were either outdated or inappropriate for specific patient cases. This wasn't just a minor setback; it put patient lives at risk and increased the burden on healthcare providers who had to double-check the algorithmic suggestions, consuming valuable time and resources. There were several issues that contributed to Epic AI's failure.

Inadequate Data

The performance of any machine learning algorithm fundamentally relies on the quality and quantity of the data. In this case, the algorithms were trained on a dataset that was either too small, poorly structured, or incomplete, reducing the reliability and generalizability of the model.

Inadequate data can lead to inaccurate predictions or misclassifications. This is especially dangerous in medical settings where lives are at stake. For example, an algorithm trained on a non-representative patient population might make incorrect or harmful recommendations for patients from underrepresented groups, thereby perpetuating healthcare disparities.

It is crucial to collect more balanced and representative datasets that account for diverse variables such as age, gender, ethnicity, and disease subtypes. Moreover, the quality of data must be rigorously assessed and validated to ensure that the algorithm's training data are both comprehensive and precise.

Lack of Clinical Input

Developing medical algorithms without the input of healthcare professionals ignores the complex reality of medical practice. Medical professionals bring insights into patient behavior, ethical considerations, and practical limitations that engineers and data scientists might overlook.

Lack of clinical input can result in algorithms that are theoretically sound but practically inapplicable or that make recommendations inconsistent with medical best practices. This can endanger patient safety and waste valuable healthcare resources.

Collaboration between engineers, data scientists, and healthcare professionals is essential from the earliest stages of development. Medical experts should be involved in data annotation, algorithm training, and validation processes to ensure that the AI system aligns with clinical needs and real-world applicability.

Overconfidence in AI

There was an inflated belief that AI algorithms were infallible and could operate without human intervention. This led to an over-reliance on AI solutions, discouraging critical evaluation of the algorithm's output.

This overconfidence resulted in missed opportunities for human oversight, reducing the quality of healthcare. When healthcare providers uncritically accept AI recommendations, it can lead to incorrect diagnoses, inappropriate treatments, and ultimately, compromised patient safety.

AI should be viewed as a tool that aids but does not replace human decision-making in healthcare. Regular audits, performance evaluations, and feedback loops should be implemented. Healthcare staff should also be trained to critically assess AI recommendations and understand the limitations and uncertainties associated with these systems.

The Lessons: A Revelation

The unfortunate shortcomings of the Epic AI initiative act as a potent revelation, not just for the developers involved but for the entire healthcare industry at large. This episode emphasizes several key lessons that are imperative for future undertakings in the domain of AI-assisted healthcare.

Robust Training Data

Quality control in data collection and curation is not just an optional step but an absolute necessity. Algorithms are only as good as the data they are trained on, and in healthcare, stakes are high, often involving life-or-death decisions.

Data governance protocols should be put in place to ensure that the data used for training is both comprehensive and accurate. This includes implementing rigorous quality control measures, like data validation and cross-referencing with clinical outcomes, to minimize errors and biases.

Multidisciplinary Involvement

The creation and implementation of AI in healthcare is a complex process that requires a synergistic effort. The involvement of data scientists and software engineers is important, but equally crucial is the role played by healthcare professionals who understand the ethics of medical practice.

A multi-disciplinary team should be constituted from the inception of the project. Regular meetings and reviews should be held to ensure that the algorithm not only functions as intended technically but is also aligned with clinical best practices and ethical guidelines.

The Resistance to Change: Challenges in Adopting AI in Healthcare

Psychological Barriers: The Fear of Job Loss

One of the most pervasive concerns that many people have about the increasing use of AI across various industries is the fear that machines will replace human jobs. This fear is not limited to the manufacturing or retail sectors but extends to high-skilled professions like healthcare as well. Doctors, nurses, and other healthcare professionals might perceive AI as a threat to their job security, leading to resistance against adopting these technologies. Many believe that the human element in healthcare is irreplaceable and cannot be mimicked by algorithms.

The hospital clerks that may be replaced by the digital data capture devices driven by AI have cause to complain. Labor organizations in other sectors have organized strikes and disrupted service provision over the loss of jobs. Some nurses and lab staff might feel they are the most likely to lose their jobs. According to the CDC, over 131 million patients visit a hospital every year, with over 18 million needing admission (Centers for Disease Control and Prevention, 2019). That averages out to just under 50,000 needing admission a day. Accounting for the trend that most hospitalizations are around holidays, even halving the number to compensate for that gives 25,000 patients on an ordinary day. This gives medical unions plenty of bargaining power to push for regulations that ensure job security for them as AI is embraced, since a strike in the healthcare industry, even for a day, can result in significant loss of life.

The Complexity Quagmire: AI is Not Plug-and-Play

Another significant concern is the inherent complexity of AI frameworks. These aren't simple tools that one can just plug in and start using; they require a degree of specialized knowledge for effective integration, management, and utilization. The average healthcare employee without specific training in data science or AI might find this complexity overwhelming. This could paradoxically make their jobs more challenging, as they now must navigate the labyrinthine intricacies of AI systems in addition to their regular duties (Ronen, 2023; Goldfarb & Teodoridis, 2022).

The Inertia of Established Procedures: Old Habits Die Hard

Healthcare is an industry steeped in tradition and established procedures. Many healthcare professionals have spent years, if not decades, mastering existing systems and practices. The introduction of AI technologies would require these experienced professionals to adapt to a new set of tools and methods. Such a seismic shift could be met with resistance, especially from those who feel they are already too invested in the current way of doing things to start anew.

A Deep-Rooted Distrust

When it comes to new technologies, fear often trumps reason. Consider aviation: Even though airplanes have the technology to practically fly themselves, the idea of boarding an aircraft with no pilot is unthinkable for most people. This sentiment extends to AI in healthcare as well. A pervasive lack of trust, fueled in part by popular culture and sci-fi tropes, acts as a significant roadblock to widespread adoption.

Given these barriers, the burden falls on healthcare organizations and policymakers to provide the necessary training and support to facilitate AI adoption. The inclusion of AI-related modules in medical education, ongoing training programs for existing staff, and perhaps most crucially, a support framework for the transitional period can go a long way in overcoming these barriers.

The Imperative of Patient Trust

Trust is a cornerstone of healthcare. Unless patients have faith in the systems used to diagnose and treat them, AI adoption will continue to lag. A study discussed in CNN and Fierce Healthcare reflects that nearly half of U.S. doctors are anxious about utilizing AI-powered software. Likewise, the Harvard Business Review mentions that despite AI's capability to outperform doctors in specific tasks, patients remain skeptical (Longoni & Morewedge, 2019; Longoni et al., 2021; Landi, 2019).

Sources for Further Reading:

[Harvard Business Review]
[CNN]
[Fierce Healthcare]

The Challenge and Opportunity of Change

The resistance to adopting AI in healthcare is fueled by a combination of psychological fears, concerns about complexity, and the inertia of established procedures. Addressing these concerns effectively is crucial for the successful integration of AI into healthcare systems. And while the challenges are significant, the potential benefits of AI—more accurate diagnoses, more effective treatments, and overall better patient care—make it imperative to confront these challenges head-on.

Exploring Further into the Sustainability of AI

The swift progression of artificial intelligence has inaugurated a novel phase of creativity and solution-finding. However, it has also ignited debates and concerns around the sustainability of AI systems. When considering the long-term viability and ethics of AI, multiple facets come into play: operational maintenance, ongoing training, and ethical governance. These aspects not only involve computational resources but also require persistent human vigilance.

Operational Sustainability

Maintaining the operational robustness of an AI system is a critical part of its sustainability. Regular updates are needed to cope with changes in the data landscape and computational requirements. Hardware must be kept up to date to match the processing needs of increasingly complex algorithms.

In the healthcare sector, for example, where AI tools are used for diagnostic and treatment plans, the need for reliable, high-performance computing is non-negotiable. Jon Moore's article on Chief Healthcare Executive highlights the substantial infrastructure required to handle the computational complexity and data volume in healthcare AI applications. Constant monitoring and regular audits of this infrastructure are indispensable for long-term viability.

Ongoing Training and Adaptation

Machine learning has the unique ability to learn and adapt over time. Despite this, it's a misconception to think that once trained, these models are set in stone. New data continually emerges, presenting situations that the model may not have encountered before. AI systems require ongoing training to accommodate new types of data and edge cases. As the Harvard Business Review article suggests, an ethics committee is essential not just for keeping AI initiatives ethical but also for providing an oversight mechanism for the ongoing training and refinement of the AI systems.

Cost Implications

There's a financial aspect to consider as well. Continually training AI systems with new data, ensuring data quality, and deploying updates are resource-intensive activities that can drive up operational costs (Landi, 2020; Luzniak, 2021).

Ethical and Security Checks

AI can be hacked, data can be corrupted, and algorithms can be biased. The sustainability of AI is not merely a question of technical maintenance but also of ethical integrity. Microsoft's vision, outlined by CNBC, focuses on transparent governance and setting parameters for what AI should and should not do. This governance involves continuous oversight by humans to identify and correct biases, ensure data privacy, and prevent unauthorized tampering (Feiner, 2023).

1. **Regular Audits and Quality Checks:** Data integrity and quality must be regularly audited to ensure that the AI system's predictions remain reliable.

2. **Ethics Committees:** As advised by the Harvard Business Review, establishing ethics committees can act as a governance body to ensure the AI system operates within agreed ethical boundaries.

3. **Cybersecurity Measures:** Considering the vulnerability of AI to hacks and unauthorized alterations, robust cybersecurity measures are crucial.

4. **Resource Allocation for Continuous Training:** Budgets must be set aside for the ongoing training of the AI models to adapt to new data and requirements.

5. **Transparency and Accountability:** Detailed logs and records of AI operations should be maintained to ensure transparency and to hold the system accountable for its actions.

6. **Public and Private Partnerships:** Collaboration between various stakeholders can help in resource pooling and sharing of best practices for the sustainable development and deployment of AI.

By focusing on these dimensions, the longevity and responsible management of AI systems can be ensured. The question, therefore, is not whether AI is sustainable but how we can make it so through concerted, ongoing efforts.

The Complex Landscape of AI Integration in Healthcare: Regulatory Compliance and Trust

As artificial intelligence makes its way into healthcare systems, it brings the promise of revolutionizing diagnostics, treatment plans, and overall patient care. However, this transformative potential comes with its own set of challenges that are unique to the healthcare ecosystem. Specifically, two critical issues stand out: the hurdles of regulatory compliance and the question of trust and acceptance from healthcare professionals and the public.

Regulatory Compliance: A Double-Edged Sword

In healthcare, where human lives are at stake, regulatory compliance is both crucial and complex. On one hand, stringent regulations are necessary to ensure that AI systems meet the highest standards of safety, efficacy, and ethics. This involves rigorous testing, validation, and ongoing audits to make sure the technology not only performs as promised but also adheres to ethical norms and respects patient confidentiality.

Just like human medical personnel, AI systems must comply with current data protection laws such as the Health Insurance Portability and Accountability Act (HIPAA) in the U.S. or the General Data Protection Regulation (GDPR) in the EU. Failure to comply can result in severe penalties and erode patient trust (Corporate Compliance Insights, 2022).

A new FDA tier has been introduced called *higher risk*. It is commonly utilized in software management that provides Clinical Decision Support (CDS). Amy Abernathy, the Principal Deputy Commissioner, explained that the higher-risk software, including advanced software that uses machine learning, can identify a patient likely to suffer from significant medical complications such as cardiovascular events or other such occurrences. Yet, it cannot explain how it made the identification, which is a problem, as patients may not be able to fully understand the AI's logic process and input parameters without additional context. The suggested legislation requires these programs to be able to both identify and explain how they made these calls (Guo et al., 2020).

AI's ability to parse through large datasets can potentially violate privacy norms if not properly contained. Striking the right balance between AI's data accessibility and patient privacy is a growing concern for regulators (Ernst and Young, 2023).

Due to the global nature of data and technology, there is a growing call for harmonized ethical and regulatory frameworks for AI in healthcare. Efforts are required at both national and international levels to make this a reality (Durgampudi, 2023).

However, these regulations also introduce a barrier to rapid innovation. Regulatory frameworks often behind technological advancements, leading to a slow, cumbersome process for AI approval and integration. This can deter investment and inhibit the agile deployment of potentially life-saving technologies.

Trust and Acceptance: A Multifaceted Issue

General Trust

Public skepticism toward AI in healthcare is not unfounded. Concerns range from the potential for misdiagnosis to data privacy issues. Moreover, as healthcare decisions carry a significant emotional weight, people may feel uneasy allowing a machine, however advanced, to make decisions that could directly impact their lives or those of their loved ones.

Physician Trust

Perhaps even more critical than general trust is the acceptance of AI by healthcare providers themselves. Physicians, who rely on years of training and a deep understanding of treating patients, may be hesitant to entrust part of their practice to an algorithm. They may question AI's capability to comprehend the complexities and variables involved in healthcare decisions, from interpreting test results to considering a patient's medical history and coexisting conditions.

Moving Forward: A Balanced Approach

Regulatory compliance in AI-driven healthcare is a multifaceted challenge that extends beyond mere adherence to existing laws. It also involves ethical considerations, robust cybersecurity, and a constant cycle of oversight and updates. Failure in any of these areas could compromise patient safety and privacy, erode trust, and ultimately hinder the broader adoption and benefits of AI in healthcare.

Successfully addressing these challenges requires a balanced approach that respects the stringent requirements of healthcare regulations while fostering an environment conducive to innovation. Alongside this, targeted efforts are needed to build trust among healthcare providers and the public. This could involve transparent reporting on the performance and limitations of AI systems, as well as ongoing education and collaboration between AI developers and healthcare professionals.

We have examined the difficulties of integrating AI in the healthcare industry. From the fear of the unknown to questions about long-term sustainability, we've dissected the issues that organizations and individuals face. Regulatory compliance stands as a formidable hurdle, especially in sensitive sectors like healthcare, where the stakes are high. As we dig deeper, the overarching theme becomes clear: The path to harnessing the full potential of AI is fraught with challenges that demand a multi-pronged, continually evolving approach.

Chapter 8:

Looking to the Future

The Promising Horizons of AI in Healthcare

In this chapter, we will examine the profound benefits and advantages of effectively integrating and managing AI within healthcare systems. Our discussion will encompass potential major enhancements in medical treatment and the viable opportunities that arise when AI is thoughtfully integrated.

As we embark on this exploration of AI in healthcare, it's crucial to understand that the greatest challenge lies not in the capabilities of AI technologies but in ensuring their seamless adoption in daily clinical practice. For widespread adoption to occur, AI systems must resolve complex issues involving regulatory approval, integration with Electronic Health Record (EHR) systems, standardization, clinician training, financial support from public or private payer organizations, and continuous field updates (Davenport & Kalakota, 2019).

AI Integration: The Possibilities

The integration of artificial intelligence in healthcare is a transformative process that can significantly improve patient outcomes, streamline healthcare services, and lower costs. Let's explore the potential applications of AI across various facets of healthcare.

For Patients

Personalized Treatment Plans: AI algorithms can analyze a patient's medical history, genomic data, and other variables to tailor treatments specifically suited to individual health profiles.

Early Detection: Machine learning models trained on vast datasets can spot anomalies in diagnostic tests much earlier than traditional methods, leading to earlier interventions.

Telehealth: AI can power chatbots that provide immediate, data-driven advice for minor healthcare concerns, thereby reducing the load on healthcare systems and offering quicker assistance to patients.

Mental Health Support: AI-driven applications can provide continual emotional support and mental health assessments, enabling better management of conditions like depression and anxiety.

For Healthcare Providers

Workflow Automation: From appointment scheduling to billing, AI can manage administrative tasks that otherwise consume a significant amount of healthcare professionals' time.

Clinical Decision Support: AI can assist doctors by providing data-driven insights during diagnosis and treatment, thereby reducing the probability of human error.

Imaging Analysis: AI algorithms can quickly and accurately analyze medical images, assisting radiologists and other specialists in their work.

Drug Discovery: AI can process complex biochemical interactions at a scale and speed unattainable for human researchers, significantly cutting the time and cost of drug development.

Out-Patient or At-Home Care

Remote Monitoring: Wearables and sensors powered by AI can monitor a patient's vitals and other health indicators in real time, alerting healthcare providers or patients themselves of any concerning changes.

Rehabilitation: AI-powered robotic arms and other devices can assist in the physical rehabilitation process, providing data on a patient's recovery and adjusting exercise regimens accordingly.

Virtual Health Assistants: For chronic conditions like diabetes or hypertension, AI can offer consistent monitoring and actionable insights right at home, allowing patients to manage their health more effectively.

Emergency Response: AI can analyze data from wearables to detect emergency situations like heart attacks, automatically alerting medical professionals and family members.

AI's role in healthcare is not without its challenges, such as data privacy concerns, the potential for algorithmic bias, and ethical considerations around decision-making. However, the potential benefits are so vast that they warrant ongoing research and implementation, with careful consideration of these issues. The integration of AI into healthcare is not just a technological evolution; it's a paradigm shift in how healthcare can be delivered and experienced.

Resolving Hurdles on the Path to AI-Enhanced Healthcare

In the previous chapters, we've explored the immense potential of AI in healthcare. Now, it's time to address the critical challenges and limitations that stand between us and the realization of this potential. In this section, we will propose practical solutions to these hurdles.

Regulatory Compliance Challenges and Proposed Solutions

Challenges

The integration of artificial intelligence into healthcare introduces a myriad of benefits, from diagnostic precision to administrative efficiency. However, a significant roadblock remains: the complex and stringent landscape of regulatory compliance. AI systems must adhere to the stringent standards established by regulatory authorities such as the U.S. Food and Drug Administration (FDA) or the European Medicines Agency (EMA), ensuring the safety of patients and the security of their data. These regulations often involve rigorous testing and validation processes, ethical considerations, and ongoing performance assessments. Non-compliance not only exposes healthcare providers to legal repercussions but also risks the safety and confidentiality of patient data.

Proposed Solutions

Clear Guidelines for AI Integration: Collaboration between healthcare organizations and regulatory bodies is critical for streamlining compliance. Both parties can work together to create guidelines that are tailored to the unique challenges and potential of AI technologies. This cooperation will lead to more efficient and clearer paths to compliance and will mitigate risks associated with the misinterpretation or misunderstanding of regulatory requirements.

Standardized AI Frameworks: A standardized framework for AI in healthcare can simplify compliance procedures by offering a consistent set of protocols and benchmarks. Healthcare providers and tech developers should advocate for these standardized systems, which can hasten the adoption of AI technologies while maintaining rigorous safety standards.

Robust Auditing and Reporting Mechanisms: To ensure ongoing compliance and performance, there must be mechanisms for auditing AI systems. These should include real-time tracking of algorithmic decisions, performance metrics, and any deviations from expected behavior. Thorough reporting should be accessible and understandable to both technical and non-technical stakeholders, providing insights that can be used to improve the AI system further.

Transparency in AI Development: Transparency in the development and deployment stages is crucial for facilitating regulatory assessments. Open dialogue about the data sources, training methodologies, and potential biases of an AI system will allow for more effective evaluations by regulatory bodies. Transparent practices also engender trust among healthcare providers and patients, fostering greater acceptance and use of AI technologies.

(Refer to the following sources for detailed insights:

<u>Source 1</u>: ComplianceNavigator

<u>Source 2</u>: Thepharmaletter

<u>Source 3</u>: Lexology

<u>Source 4</u>: Inmoment

Cost and Accessibility Challenges and Proposed Solutions

Challenges

The implementation of artificial intelligence in healthcare, although promising, comes with its set of challenges related to cost and accessibility. Advanced AI solutions often require substantial investments in technology, data analytics, training, and ongoing maintenance. These costs can be prohibitive for many healthcare organizations, particularly smaller ones with limited budgets. Furthermore, there's the critical issue of accessibility; the benefits of AI should not be confined to well-funded urban centers but must be available to all, including rural and underserved communities. Failing to address this can exacerbate existing healthcare inequalities, creating a two-tiered system where only the affluent have access to the best AI-powered healthcare services.

Proposed Solutions

Cost-Effective AI Solutions: One approach to mitigate the cost barrier is to explore more affordable AI platforms. Open-source AI platforms can significantly reduce upfront costs by offering foundational algorithms and tools that organizations can build upon. Cloud-based services also provide a scalable option that avoids the need for large initial investments in hardware and other infrastructure.

Partnerships for Shared Infrastructure Costs: Healthcare organizations can collaborate with AI solution providers, or even other healthcare institutions, to share the costs of infrastructure and implementation. Through partnerships, organizations can pool resources for mutual benefit, sharing data storage solutions, computing power, and even personnel trained in AI technologies. These partnerships can accelerate the adoption of AI by making it financially feasible for more organizations.

Government Initiatives for Underserved Communities: To improve accessibility, healthcare organizations can advocate for government policies that specifically bring AI technologies to underserved areas. Grants, tax incentives, and public-private partnerships can stimulate investment in healthcare AI for rural and disadvantaged communities. State and federal initiatives can also fund research into how AI can be adapted to meet the unique healthcare challenges faced by these populations.

Telehealth and Remote Solutions: For areas where healthcare facilities are sparse, AI-powered telehealth solutions can be a boon. These services can provide crucial healthcare access to distant or isolated communities at a fraction of the cost of building and staffing new facilities.

(Refer to the following sources for cost-effective strategies:

    <u>Source 1</u>: **Builtin**

    <u>Source 2</u>: **Forbes**

    <u>Source 3</u>: **ScienceDirect**

Trust and Adoption Challenges and the Proposed Solutions

Challenges

For AI technologies to truly revolutionize healthcare, trust and widespread adoption are indispensable. Both healthcare providers and patients often harbor skepticism and concerns about the reliability, accuracy, and ethical implications of AI. This lack of trust can be a significant roadblock to the integration of AI solutions in healthcare settings. Doctors may hesitate to rely on AI-driven diagnostic tools or treatment plans, while patients may question the confidentiality and precision of AI-powered services. Therefore, strategies to build and sustain trust are pivotal for the successful rollout and long-term efficacy of healthcare AI.

Proposed Solutions

AI Education and Training Programs: A lack of understanding often fuels skepticism. Healthcare professionals may be more likely to trust AI if they understand its capabilities and limitations. Targeted education and training programs can demystify AI technologies, providing healthcare workers with the knowledge they need to use these tools effectively. These programs should not only cover the technical aspects but also address the ethical and practical considerations related to AI in healthcare.

Transparent Algorithms: One of the challenges in building trust is the *black box* nature of many AI algorithms, which make decisions that users can't easily understand or explain. Developing AI algorithms that are transparent and provide understandable explanations for their decisions can alleviate these concerns. Explainable AI (XAI) models can help both doctors and patients feel more comfortable by offering insights into how a particular healthcare outcome was reached.

Sharing Success Stories: Nothing builds confidence like success. Healthcare organizations should be encouraged to share case studies and success stories that showcase the positive outcomes generated by AI. These could range from faster and more accurate diagnoses to efficient administrative procedures that provide more time for patient care. Publicizing these achievements can serve as tangible evidence of AI's potential benefits, thereby bolstering trust among healthcare providers and patients alike.

Patient Engagement and Feedback: Directly involving patients in the AI adoption process can also build trust. By gathering and acting on feedback from patients who have experienced AI-driven healthcare services, organizations can not only improve these services but also demonstrate a commitment to patient-centered care, further fostering trust.

Third-Party Reviews and Certifications: Another way to build trust is through external validation. Healthcare organizations can seek third-party reviews or certifications for their AI solutions, offering an unbiased perspective on their reliability and efficacy.

Refer to the following sources for strategies to enhance trust and adoption:

<u>Source 1</u>: **Entrepreneur**

<u>Source 2</u>: **Healthcare IT News**

<u>Source 3</u>: **ScienceDirect**

Conclusion:

The Future of AI in Healthcare—A Revolution in the Making

The Unmistakable Message

In traversing the terrain of AI integration in healthcare through the pages of this book, it's evident that the realm of possibilities is both expansive and exhilarating. While the book doesn't claim to be an exhaustive exploration of every facet, the resounding message across the chapters is unmistakable: AI isn't just another tool in the healthcare toolbox—it's a transformative force that holds the promise of redefining healthcare delivery.

The Key Takeaway: A Beacon of Hope and Change

AI stands as more than just a technological advancement; it's a beacon of hope for an industry that faces increasing challenges, from aging populations to burgeoning healthcare costs. It has the power to turn the tide by enabling more accurate diagnoses, personalized treatments tailored to individual patient needs, and a holistic approach to patient care that enhances both efficiency and outcomes. The beauty lies in the marriage of human expertise and AI's computational prowess, a synergy that has the potential to usher in an unprecedented era of healthcare excellence.

Success Stories: Where Innovation Meets Impact

Throughout our journey, we've touched upon compelling narratives of transformative success. From AI algorithms that can detect life-threatening diseases at stages so early that they were previously undetectable to robotic assistants that aid in complex surgeries with a level of precision previously thought unattainable, the stories are awe-inspiring. AI has even started to impact mental health care, providing timely insights and interventions. These successes are not merely isolated instances but serve as concrete proof that, when leveraged correctly, AI can lead to breakthroughs that redefine the boundaries of what we deem possible in healthcare.

The Ethical and Social Dimensions: Balancing Innovation and Responsibility

It would be remiss not to acknowledge the complex ethical and social dimensions that accompany AI's integration. Issues such as data privacy, equitable access, and algorithmic fairness pose important questions. The book has discussed how the healthcare industry, along with regulatory bodies, are taking diligent steps to guide themselves and each other through these challenges, striving for a future where AI serves as a tool for good, available and beneficial to all.

A Call to Action: The Crossroads of Opportunity and Responsibility

As we close this chapter and consider the road ahead, we find ourselves standing at a crucial crossroads. With the comprehensive insights gained, we can no longer afford to be passive observers. The understanding of both the enormous potential and the very real challenges AI presents provides us with the responsibility to act. It is up to healthcare professionals, technologists, policymakers, and indeed all of us as stakeholders in global health to ensure that AI is implemented in ways that are safe, ethical, and equitable.

In summary, the horizon of AI in healthcare is expansive and full of promise yet laden with challenges that require collective wisdom and action. As we forge ahead, it's crucial to maintain a balanced perspective that is as cautious as it is optimistic. The concerted efforts of everyone involved can turn the promise of AI in healthcare into a tangible reality, elevating the standard of care to heights previously unimaginable.

A Note to Our Valued Readers

Dear Reader,

First and foremost, thank you for journeying through the pages of this book. I truly hope it provided insights, knowledge, and perhaps even a fresh perspective on AI in healthcare.

Your feedback means the world to me. It not only informs future works but also help other readers make informed choices. If you found this book insightful, engaging, or beneficial in any way, I'd be honored if you could take a few minutes to share your experiences and thoughts by leaving a review.

[Insert Link to Review Platform, if applicable]

Here's how:

Visit [Review Platform Name, e.g., Amazon/Goodreads].

Locate this book by searching for *Transforming Healthcare: Harnessing the Power of Artificial Intelligence for Enhanced Patient Care* by SB Wade.

Click on *Write a Review* or a similar option.

Share your thoughts and rate the book based on your experience.

Every review, whether it's detailed or succinct, contributes to my continuous journey of growth and refinement. Moreover, your feedback helps guide fellow readers on their literary journey.

Thank you once again for choosing to read this book and for considering sharing your reflections. Your support is invaluable to me and the broader community of readers.

Warm regards,

SB Wade

Glossary

Definition of terms according to MITA (Medical Imaging and Technology Alliance) a division of NEMA

- **Algorithms (Clustering, Classification, Regression, and Recommendation)**: A set of rules or instructions given to an AI, neural network, or other machine to help it learn on its own.

- **Analytical Validation**: The measure of the ability of a task to accurately and reliably generate the intended technical output from the input data.

- **Artificial Neural Network (ANN)**: A learning model created to act like a human brain that solves tasks that are too difficult for traditional computer systems to solve.

- **Artificial Intelligence (AI)**: Refers to the simulation of human intelligence in machines that can perform tasks, learn from experience, and make autonomous decisions.

- **Augmented Intelligence, also known as Intelligence Augmentation (IA)**: Systems that are designed to enhance human capabilities. This is contrasted with Artificial Intelligence, which is intended to replicate or replace human intelligence.

- **Augmented Reality (AR)**: Technology that overlays digital information or virtual objects onto the real-world environment, enhancing the user's perception and interaction with their surroundings.

- **Bias in AI**: The presence of systematic favoritism or discrimination in AI algorithms, leading to differential treatment or outcomes for certain patient groups.

- **Chatbot**: A program that is designed to simulate a conversation with human users by communicating through text chats, voice commands, or both. They are a commonly used interface for computer programs that include AI capabilities.

- **Classification**: The problem of identifying to which of a set of categories (sub-populations) a new observation belongs on the basis of a training set of data containing observations (or instances) whose category membership is known.

- **Clinical Decision Support System (CDSS)**: AI-based systems that provide healthcare professionals with evidence-based recommendations and alerts to support clinical decision-making.

- **Clustering**: Algorithms that let machines group data points or items into groups with similar characteristics.

- **Cognitive Computing**: A computerized model that mimics the way the human brain thinks. It involves self-learning through the use of data mining, natural language processing, and pattern recognition.

- **Computer-Aided Detection (CADe)**: Refers to pattern recognition software that identifies suspicious features on the image and brings them to the attention of the radiologist in order to decrease false negative readings.

- **Computer-Aided Diagnosis (CADx)**: Refers to software that analyzes a radiographic finding to estimate the likelihood that the feature represents a specific disease process (e.g., benign versus malignant).

- **Computer Vision**: A field of AI that enables computers to understand and interpret visual information from images or videos.

- **Convolutional Neural Network (CNN)**: A type of neural network that identifies and makes sense of images.

- **Continuous Learning Systems (CLS)**: Systems that are inherently capable of learning from real-world data and are able to update themselves automatically over time while in public use.

- **Data Mining**: The examination of data sets to discover patterns from that data that can be of further use.

- **Data Privacy and Security**: The protection of sensitive patient information and healthcare data from unauthorized access, breaches, or misuse.

- **Deep Learning**: A subfield of ML that uses artificial neural networks to model and understand complex patterns and relationships in data.

- **Electronic Health Record (EHR)**: Digital records that contain a patient's medical history, including diagnoses, treatments, medications, and laboratory results.

- **Explainable AI**: The ability of AI systems to provide transparent and interpretable explanations for their decisions or predictions, enabling users to understand the underlying reasoning and build trust.

- **False Negative**: Test result that does not detect the condition when the condition is present.

- **False Positive**: Test result that detects the condition when the condition is absent.

- **Genetic Algorithm**: An evolutionary algorithm based on principles of genetics and natural selection that is used to find optimal or near-optimal solutions to difficult problems that would otherwise take decades to solve.

- **Heuristic Search Techniques**: Support that narrows down the search to optimal solutions for a problem by eliminating options that are incorrect.

- **Historical Control Clinical Trial**: A type of clinical trial where the percentage change in disease detection and recall/workup rates is determined by comparing data before and after the implementation of CAD into clinical practice.

- **Internet of Medical Things (IoMT)**: The network of medical devices, wearables, and sensors connected to the internet, enabling the collection and sharing of healthcare data for analysis and decision-making.

- **Knowledge Engineering**: Engineering focused on building knowledge-based systems, including all of the scientific, technical, and social aspects of it.

- **Machine Learning (ML)**: A subset of AI that focuses on the development of algorithms and models that enable systems to learn and make predictions or decisions without explicit programming.

- **Machine Perception**: The ability of a system to receive and interpret data from the outside world, similar to how humans use their senses. This is typically done with attached hardware, such as sensors.

- **Natural Language Processing (NLP)**: The ability of machines to understand and process human language, enabling applications like voice recognition and language translation.

- **Pattern Recognition**: A branch of machine learning that focuses on the recognition of patterns and regularities in data, although it is in some cases considered to be nearly synonymous with machine learning.

- **Precision Medicine**: An approach to healthcare that tailors medical treatment and interventions to individual patients based on their unique characteristics, including genetic information and personal health data.

- **Predictive Analytics**: The use of AI and statistical modeling techniques to analyze historical data and make predictions about future outcomes or events.

- **Real-Time Health Systems (RTHS)**: Information systems that collect and analyze real-time information from a patient; in contrast to systems that take a patient's blood pressure or heart rate only when they are in the doctor's office or admitted to a hospital.

- **Recommendation Algorithms**: Algorithms that help machines suggest a choice based on its commonality with historical data.

- **Recurrent Neural Network (RNN)**: A type of neural network that makes sense of sequential information and recognizes patterns, and creates outputs based on those calculations.

- **Regression**: A statistical approach that helps predict future outcomes or items in a continuous data set by solving for the pattern of past inputs, such as linear regression in statistics. Regression is foundational to machine learning and artificial intelligence.

- **Reinforcement Learning**: A type of machine learning where algorithms are trained through interactions with an environment. When an algorithm's processes deliver desired results, it receives positive feedback. For example, the algorithm receives a reward for scoring a point or winning a game.

- **Remote Patient Monitoring**: The use of connected devices and AI to collect and monitor patient health data remotely, enabling continuous monitoring and early detection of health issues.

- **Sequential Read Clinical Trial**: A clinical trial where the exam is first read prior to, and then following, CAD input. The change in disease detection due to the CAD input, as well as the change in the recall/workup rates, will determine the contribution of CAD to patient management. Importantly, the percentage increase in disease detection should be concordant with, or less than, the percentage increase in the recall/workup rates.

- **Supervised Machine Learning**: The machine learning task of learning a function that maps an input to an output based on example input-output pairs. It infers a function from labeled training data consisting of a set of training examples.

- **True Negative**: Test result that does not detect the condition when the condition is absent.

- **True Positive**: Test result that detects the condition when the condition is present.

References

Abbasi, J. (2022). *Pushed to their limits, 1 in 5 physicians intends to leave practice.* JAMA. https://doi.org/10.1001/jama.2022.5074

Admin, H. M. G. (2020, August 12). *Is there a limit to how many patients a physician can treat?* UHC Solutions. https://www.uhcsolutions.com/is-there-a-limit-to-how-many-patients-a-physician-can-treat/

Agency for Healthcare Research and Quality. (2018). *Data sources for health care quality measures.* Agency for Healthcare Research and Quality. https://www.ahrq.gov/talkingquality/measures/understand/index.html

Ahuja, A. S. (2019). The impact of artificial intelligence in medicine on the future role of the physician. *PeerJ*, 7. https://doi.org/10.7717/peerj.7702

AI is fast addressing data requirements and advancing interoperability, says one expert. (2022, December 27). Healthcare IT News. https://www.healthcareitnews.com/news/ai-fast-addressing-data-requirements-and-advancing-interoperability-says-one-expert

AlZaabi, A., AlMaskari, S., & AalAbdulsalam, A. (2023). Are physicians and medical students ready for artificial intelligence applications in healthcare? *Digital Health*, 9. https://doi.org/10.1177/20552076231152167

Andreotta, A. J., Kirkham, N., & Rizzi, M. (2021). AI, big data, and the future of consent. *AI & Society*, 37. https://doi.org/10.1007/s00146-021-01262-5

Bartels, R., Dudink, J., Haitjema, S., Oberski, D., & van 't Veen, A. (2022). A Perspective on a Quality Management System for AI/ML-Based Clinical Decision Support in Hospital Care.

Frontiers in Digital Health, 4. https://doi.org/10.3389/fdgth.2022.942588

Bartley, J. (2014, August 30). *The benefits and limits of technology in medical practices.* Physicians Practice. https://www.physicianspractice.com/view/benefits-and-limits-technology-medical-practices

Basu, K., Sinha, R., Ong, A., & Basu, T. (2020). Artificial Intelligence: How is it changing medical sciences and its future? *Indian Journal of Dermatology,* 65(5), 365–370. https://doi.org/10.4103/ijd.IJD_421_20

Bawa, A. (2021, March 5). *This Singapore based startup uses artificial intelligence powered clinical assistant to improve doctor's productivity and patient care.* MarkTechPost. https://www.marktechpost.com/2021/03/05/this-singapore-based-startup-uses-artificial-intelligence-powered-clinical-assistant-to-improve-doctors-productivity-and-patient-care/

Bawa, A., & Bawa, A. (2022, September 19). *14 real-world applications of artificial intelligence (AI) in the healthcare industry.* MarkTechPost. https://www.marktechpost.com/2022/09/18/14-real-world-applications-of-artificial-intelligence-ai-in-the-healthcare-industry/

Bestsennyy, O., & Cordina, J. (2021, August 5). *Role of personalization in the care journey.* McKinsey. https://www.mckinsey.com/industries/healthcare/our-insights/the-role-of-personalization-in-the-care-journey-an-example-of-patient-engagement-to-reduce-readmissions

Biotech begins human trials with drug discovered using AI. (2022, October 31). Financial Times. https://www.ft.com/content/0006ae3f-7064-4aa6-98cd-8912f544acc5

Bresko, D. K. M. G. (2023, April 17). *Healthcare analytics and AI large language model.* Cerner. https://www.cerner.com/ae/en/blog/healthcare-analytics-and-ai-large-language-model

Breus, M. J. (2011, July 26). *New limits on resident physicians' hours—do they go far enough?* Psychology Today. https://www.psychologytoday.com/us/blog/sleep-newzzz/201107/new-limits-on-resident-physicians-hours-do-they-go-far-enough

Brocollo, B., & Peregrine, M. (2022, February 9). *AI Could Be the Magic Pill for Improved Health Care, but Ethical Concerns Are a Side-Effect.* Corporate Compliance Insights. https://www.corporatecomplianceinsights.com/ai-health-care-regulators-boards-laws-ethical-concerns/

Brown, S. (2021, April 21). *Machine learning, explained.* MIT Sloan School of Management. https://mitsloan.mit.edu/ideas-made-to-matter/machine-learning-explained

Campbell, D. (2017, November 27). *Hospital patients complain of rude staff, lack of compassion and long waits.* The Guardian. https://www.theguardian.com/society/2011/feb/23/hospital-patients-rude-staff-long-waits

Capone, A. (2022, January 11). *The future of healthcare technology.* Forbes. https://www.forbes.com/sites/forbestechcouncil/2022/01/11/the-future-of-healthcare-technology/?sh=737c8d614750

Chambers, N. (2019, January 22). *Our children's career aspirations have nothing in common with the jobs of the future.* World Economic Forum. https://www.weforum.org/agenda/2019/01/childrens-career-aspirations-jobs-of-future/

Christensen, J. (2023, February 22). *Most Americans are uncomfortable with artificial intelligence in health care, survey finds.* CNN.

https://edition.cnn.com/2023/02/22/health/artificial-intelligence-health-care/index.html

Cohen, G. (2020). Informed Consent and Medical Artificial Intelligence: What to Tell the Patient? *The Georgetown Law Journal,* 6. https://www.law.georgetown.edu/georgetown-law-journal/in-print/volume-108/volume-108-issue-6-june-2020/informed-consent-and-medical-artificial-intelligence-what-to-tell-the-patient/

Davenport, T., & Kalakota, R. (2019). The potential for artificial intelligence in healthcare. *Future Healthcare Journal,* 6(2), 94–98. https://doi.org/10.7861/futurehosp.6-2-94

Dettling, H. U., Jacobus, K., & Wassen, D. T. (2021, July 21). *How the challenge of regulating AI in healthcare is escalating.* EY. https://www.ey.com/en_gl/law/how-the-challenge-of-regulating-ai-in-healthcare-is-escalating

Dunlap, S. (2022, March 10). *5 examples of smart technology in healthcare.* Impact Networking. https://www.impactmybiz.com/blog/smart-technology-in-healthcare/

Editorial Team. (2022, October 5). *Top 10 Medical Technologies 2022: Innovations In The Medical Field.* Tech Business News. https://www.techbusinessnews.com.au/top-10-medical-technologies-2022-innovations-in-the-medical-field/

Farhud, D. D., & Zokaei, S. (2021). Ethical Issues of Artificial Intelligence in Medicine and Healthcare. *Iranian Journal of Public Health,* 50(11). https://doi.org/10.18502/ijph.v50i11.7600

Feiner, L. (2023, May 25). *Microsoft outlines its vision for keeping A.I. in check.* CNBC. https://www.cnbc.com/2023/05/25/microsoft-outlines-its-vision-for-keeping-ai-in-check.html

Feng, J., Phillips, R. V., Malenica, I., Bishara, A., Hubbard, A. E., Celi, L. A., & Pirracchio, R. (2022). Clinical artificial intelligence quality improvement: towards continual monitoring and updating of AI algorithms in healthcare. *Npj Digital Medicine, 5*(1). https://doi.org/10.1038/s41746-022-00611-y

Forbes Technology Council. (2017, April 18). *Seven Affordable Ways To Incorporate Machine Learning And AI Into Your Business.* Forbes. https://www.forbes.com/sites/forbestechcouncil/2018/04/17/seven-affordable-ways-to-incorporate-machine-learning-and-ai-into-your-business/?sh=69895a554baf

Four ways AI can make healthcare more efficient and affordable. (2018, May 31). World Economic Forum. https://medium.com/world-economic-forum/four-ways-ai-can-make-healthcare-more-efficient-and-affordable-85957e34944f

Fox, A. (2022, September 15). *Developing trust in healthcare AI, step by step.* Healthcare IT News. https://www.healthcareitnews.com/news/developing-trust-healthcare-ai-step-step

Genomics. (2015). Office of Science. https://www.energy.gov/science/genomics

Goetz, L. H., & Schork, N. J. (2018). Personalized medicine: motivation, challenges, and progress. *Fertility and Sterility, 109*(6), 952–963. https://doi.org/10.1016/j.fertnstert.2018.05.006

Goldfarb, A., & Teodoridis, F. (2022, March 9). *Why is AI adoption in health care lagging?* Brookings. https://www.brookings.edu/articles/why-is-ai-adoption-in-health-care-lagging/

Grissinger, M. (2017). Disrespectful Behavior in Health Care: Its Impact, Why It Arises and Persists, And How to Address It-

Part 2. *P & T: A Peer-Reviewed Journal for Formulary Management,* *42*(2), 74–77. https://www.ncbi.nlm.nih.gov/pmc/articles/PMC5265230/

Guilliams, T. (2022, May 5). *The Ethical Adoption Of AI In Healthcare Requires A Global Effort, Now More Than Ever.* Forbes. https://www.forbes.com/sites/forbestechcouncil/2022/05/05/the-ethical-adoption-of-ai-in-healthcare-requires-a-global-effort-now-more-than-ever/?sh=6298fa1e612a

Habli, I., Lawton, T., & Porter, Z. (2020). Artificial intelligence in health care: accountability and safety. *Bulletin of the World Health Organization,* *98*(4), 251–256. https://doi.org/10.2471/blt.19.237487

Harvard Business Review. (2014, August 1). *Technology and human vulnerability.* Harvard Business Review. https://hbr.org/2003/09/technology-and-human-vulnerability

Hayes, E. (2021, May 28). *The importance of fully interoperable healthcare systems.* Forbes. https://www.forbes.com/sites/forbestechcouncil/2021/05/28/the-importance-of-fully-interoperable-healthcare-systems/?sh=235330aa230e

Heredi-Szabo, G. (2022, September 12). *Moxa medical application devices.* KnowHow. https://knowhow.distrelec.com/medical-healthcare/moxa-medical-application-devices/

HIMSS. (2020, August 4). *Interoperability in healthcare.* HIMSS. https://www.himss.org/resources/interoperability-healthcare#Part1

History of Healthcare in Canada - 1914-1929 - Canadian Hospitals. (2010, March 31). Canada Museum of History. https://www.historymuseum.ca/cmc/exhibitions/hist/medicare/medic-1c02e.html

Hogg, R., Hanley, J., & Smith, P. (2018). Learning lessons from the analysis of patient complaints relating to staff attitudes, behaviour and communication, using the concept of emotional labour. *Journal of Clinical Nursing, 27*(5-6), e1004–e1012. https://doi.org/10.1111/jocn.14121

Huded, C., Rosno, J., & Prasad, V. (2013). When research evidence is misleading. *AMA Journal of Ethics, 15*(1), 29–33. https://doi.org/10.1001/virtualmentor.2013.15.1.jdsc1-1301.

Impact of delay in care a common reason for complaints, health watchdog says. (2023, April 28). RNZ. https://www.rnz.co.nz/news/national/488844/impact-of-delay-in-care-a-common-reason-for-complaints-health-watchdog-says

Insider Intelligence Team. (2022, April 15). *Use of AI in healthcare & medicine is booming – here's how the medical field is benefiting from AI in 2022 and beyond.* Insider Intelligence. https://www.insiderintelligence.com/insights/artificial-intelligence-healthcare/

Interoperability in healthcare. (n.d.). IBM. https://www.ibm.com/topics/interoperability-in-healthcare

Interoperability in healthcare: Type, and benefits. (n.d.). PatientMD. https://patientmd.com/blogs/interoperability-in-healthcare-type-and-benefits-aX4rERZz

Ioannidis, J. P. A. (2005). Why Most Published Research Findings Are False. *PLoS Medicine, 2*(8), e124. https://doi.org/10.1371/journal.pmed.0020124

Janvier, J. (2021, September 1). *Why is interoperability important in healthcare?* Audacious Inquiry. https://ainq.com/why-is-interoperability-important-in-healthcare/

Jennings, K. (2020, October 28). *How human genome sequencing went from $1 Billion A pop to under $1,000.* Forbes.

https://www.forbes.com/sites/katiejennings/2020/10/28/how-human-genome-sequencing-went-from-1-billion-a-pop-to-under-1000/?sh=46acf4ae8cea

Johnson, V. (2020, May 19). *Why can't I be tested for ALL sexually transmitted infections?* Planned Parenthood. https://www.plannedparenthood.org/planned-parenthood-st-louis-region-southwest-missouri/blog/why-cant-i-be-tested-for-all-sexually-transmitted-infections

KDnuggets. (2023, April 28). *Introducing healthcare-specific Large Language Models from John Snow labs.* KDnuggets. https://www.kdnuggets.com/2023/04/john-snow-introducing-healthcare-specific-large-language-models-john-snow-labs.html

Kickstart your design. (2023). Visily. https://www.visily.ai/

Kaplan, S. (2022, September 1). *Successes and Failures of U.S. Space Launch.* Aerospace Security. https://aerospace.csis.org/data/u-s-space-launch-success-and-failure/

Klass, P., & M.d. (2017, April 10). *Rude Doctors, Rude Nurses, Rude Patients.* The New York Times. https://www.nytimes.com/2017/04/10/well/family/rude-doctors-rude-nurses-rude-patients.html

Kuan, R. (2019, October 18). *Adopting AI in Health Care Will Be Slow and Difficult.* Harvard Business Review. https://hbr.org/2019/10/adopting-ai-in-health-care-will-be-slow-and-difficult

Kuhn, J. (2023, June 20). *AI and Large Language Models: The future of healthcare data interoperability.* Forbes. https://www.forbes.com/sites/forbestechcouncil/2023/06/20/ai-and-large-language-models-the-future-of-healthcare-data-interoperability/?sh=4a287f9c67dc

Landi, H. (2019, April 25). *Nearly half of U.S. doctors say they are anxious about using AI-powered software: survey*. Fierce Healthcare. https://www.fiercehealthcare.com/practices/nearly-half-u-s-doctors-say-they-are-anxious-about-using-ai-powered-software-survey

Landi, H. (2020, February 19). *Healthcare CEOs say AI progress stymied by high costs, privacy risks*. Fierce Healthcare. https://www.fiercehealthcare.com/tech/artificial-intelligence-increasing-patient-access-to-care-but-it-s-also-driving-up-cost

Lehne, M., Sass, J., Essenwanger, A., Schepers, J., & Thun, S. (2019). Why digital medicine depends on interoperability. *Npj Digital Medicine, 2*(1). https://doi.org/10.1038/s41746-019-0158-1

Leibert, F. (2018, August 15). *AI will improve healthcare and cut costs - if we get these 4 things right*. World Economic Forum. https://www.weforum.org/agenda/2018/08/ai-will-improve-healthcare-and-cut-costs-of-we-get-this-right/?DAG=3&gclid=Cj0KCQjwk96lBhDHARIsAEKO4xYaKiL7MV3sZSd-LhZCqP11VwAyOknIcFXRXkpAiBRSQvceQRr-M6UaAh6WEALw_wcB

Lovell, T. (2021, July 28). *WHO warns about the risks of AI for healthcare*. Healthcare IT News. https://www.healthcareitnews.com/news/emea/who-warns-about-risks-ai-healthcare

Machine Learning Masters the Fingerprint SEP to Fool Biometric Systems. (2018, November 20). NYU Tandon School of Engineering. https://engineering.nyu.edu/news/machine-learning-masters-fingerprint-fool-biometric-systems

Malouf, W. (2015, March 3). *Recognizing the limits of a physician's work life*. Albert Einstein College of Medicine.

https://blogs.einsteinmed.edu/recognizing-the-limits-of-a-physicians-work-life/

Maloy, C. (2021). *Data resources in the health sciences: Clinical data.* Health Sciences Library University of Washington. https://guides.lib.uw.edu/hsl/data/findclin

Management of health records. (2019, October 4). CDC. https://www.cdc.gov/infectioncontrol/guidelines/healthcare-personnel/health-records.html

Mangan, D. (2015, December 4). *Personalized medicine: Better results, but at what cost?* CNBC. https://www.cnbc.com/2015/12/04/personalized-medicine-better-results-but-at-what-cost.html

Manning, C. (2020). *Artificial Intelligence Definitions.* Stanford University. https://hai.stanford.edu/sites/default/files/2020-09/AI-Definitions-HAI.pdf

Marr, B. (2022, September 22). *How AI and Machine Learning will impact the future of Healthcare.* Forbes. https://www.forbes.com/sites/bernardmarr/2022/09/14/how-ai-and-machine-learning-will-impact-the-future-of-healthcare/?sh=1ac19cc647c5

McCarthy, J. (2007). *What is Artificial Intellignece?* Formal Reasoning Group. https://www-formal.stanford.edu/jmc/whatisai.pdf

McKendrick, J. (n.d.). *Healthcare May Be The Ultimate Proving Ground For Artificial Intelligence.* Forbes. https://www.forbes.com/sites/joemckendrick/2023/02/22/healthcare-may-be-the-ultimate-proving-ground-for-artificial-intelligence/?sh=7a7c1d322b55

Mckinsey and Company. (2023, April 24). *What is AI?* McKinsey. https://www.mckinsey.com/featured-insights/mckinsey-explainers/what-is-ai

Mesko, B. (2018, May 24). *5 Reasons Why Artificial Intelligence Won't Replace Physicians*. The Medical Futurist. https://medicalfuturist.com/5-reasons-artificial-intelligence-wont-replace-physicians/

Mills, T. (2022, February 16). *AI for health and hope: How machine learning is being used in hospitals*. Forbes. https://www.forbes.com/sites/forbestechcouncil/2022/02/16/ai-for-health-and-hope-how-machine-learning-is-being-used-in-hospitals/?sh=5861d6ec55be

Moore, J. (2023, March 10). *Managing the benefits and risks of AI in healthcare*. Chief Healthcare Executive. https://www.chiefhealthcareexecutive.com/view/managing-the-benefits-and-risks-of-ai-in-healthcare-jon-moore

Nagy, M., & Sisk, B. (2020). How Will Artificial Intelligence Affect Patient-Clinician Relationships? *AMA Journal of Ethics, 22*(5), 395–400. https://doi.org/10.1001/amajethics.2020.395.

Nebergall, J. (2021, July 23). *Tackling the healthcare interoperability dilemma with artificial intelligence*. Modern Healthcare. https://www.modernhealthcare.com/information-technology/tackling-healthcare-interoperability-dilemma-artificial-intelligence

Ng, A. (2016, August 7). *IBM's Watson gives proper diagnosis for Japanese leukemia patient after doctors were stumped for months*. Daily News. https://www.nydailynews.com/news/world/ibm-watson-proper-diagnosis-doctors-stumped-article-1.2741857

Panner, M. (2019, September 4). *Personalized Medicine: The Trend That's Sweeping Health Care*. Forbes. https://www.forbes.com/sites/forbestechcouncil/2019/09/04/personalized-medicine-the-trend-thats-sweeping-health-care/?sh=581353d15444

Pearl, R. M.D. (n.d.). *Will Generative AI Wreck Or Rekindle The Doctor-Patient Relationship?* Forbes.

https://www.forbes.com/sites/robertpearl/2023/05/08/wil
l-chatgpt-wreck-or-rekindle-the-doctor-patient-
relationship/?sh=67580f1b7b81

Pocock, K. (2023, January 23). *What is Chat GPT?* PC Guide.
https://www.pcguide.com/apps/what-is-chat-gpt/

Powell, A. (2020, November 11). *Risks and benefits of an AI revolution in medicine.* Harvard Gazette.
https://news.harvard.edu/gazette/story/2020/11/risks-and-
benefits-of-an-ai-revolution-in-medicine/

Price, G., & Norbeck, T. (2018, July 18). *Physicians are human too.* Forbes.
https://www.forbes.com/sites/physiciansfoundation/2018/
07/18/physicians-are-human-too/?sh=294a59754a29

Pros & Cons of Artificial Intelligence in Medicine. (2021, July 21). Drexel University College of Computing & Informatics.
https://drexel.edu/cci/stories/artificial-intelligence-in-
medicine-pros-and-cons/

Ravinder, P. (2023, May 9). *The rise of AI: Is it the most influential invention ever?* Innovation News Network.
https://www.innovationnewsnetwork.com/rise-of-ai-most-
influential-invention-ever/32458/

Reader, T. W., Gillespie, A., & Roberts, J. (2014). Patient Complaints in Healthcare systems: a Systematic Review and Coding Taxonomy. *BMJ Quality & Safety, 23*(8), 678–689.
https://doi.org/10.1136/bmjqs-2013-002437

Ronen, O. (2023, May 9). *Obstacles To Widespread Adoption of AI in the Healthcare Industry.* Spiceworks.
https://www.spiceworks.com/tech/innovation/guest-
article/obstacles-of-ai-in-healthcare-industry/

Rosario, C. (2020, January 8). *5 benefits of interoperability in healthcare.* Advanced Data Systems Corporation.

https://www.adsc.com/blog/benefits-of-interoperability-in-healthcare

Rosen, H. (2023a, February 7). *Top Five Opportunities And Challenges Of AI In Healthcare*. Forbes. https://www.forbes.com/sites/forbesbusinesscouncil/2023/02/07/top-five-opportunities-and-challenges-of-ai-in-healthcare/?sh=2b87bdbb2805

Rosen, H. (2023b, April). *How Generative AI Can Improve Personalized Healthcare With Wearable Devices*. Forbes. https://www.forbes.com/sites/forbesbusinesscouncil/2023/04/14/how-generative-ai-can-improve-personalized-healthcare-with-wearable-devices/?sh=3639c740a3c9

Ross, C. (2021, July 26). *Epic's AI algorithms, shielded from scrutiny by a corporate firewall, are delivering inaccurate information on seriously ill patients*. STAT. https://www.statnews.com/2021/07/26/epic-hospital-algorithms-sepsis-investigation/?utm_campaign=stat_plus_today&utm_medium=email&_hsmi=143907479&_hsenc=p2ANqtz-8GWuvAgo9uiPOj583cPOE8plPk02eCtAY_IOjpX6L7lA_N7cU7kAqmVYe1aniM6yS9B2YNbsaofJLDzi2F9Imjw1IrhQ&utm_content=143907479&utm_source=hs_email

Sæther, S. M. M., Heggestad, T., Heimdal, J.-H., & Myrtveit, M. (2019). Long Waiting Times for Elective Hospital Care – Breaking the Vicious Circle by Abandoning Prioritisation. *International Journal of Health Policy and Management, 9*(3), 96–107. https://doi.org/10.15171/ijhpm.2019.84

Safani, E. (2018, September 2). *We're doctors, but we're humans too.* KevinMD. https://www.kevinmd.com/2018/09/were-doctors-but-were-humans-too.html

Schork, N. J. (2019). Artificial Intelligence and Personalized Medicine. Precision *Medicine in Cancer Therapy*, 265–283. https://doi.org/10.1007/978-3-030-16391-4_11

Senior, E. C. (2023, June 27). *Rise of the robot receptionist: AI will be used to book appointments.* Mail Online. https://www.dailymail.co.uk/health/article-12237655/Rise-robot-receptionist-AI-tech-used-schedule-appointments.html

Shrivastav, S. (2017, Apr 10). *Interning doctor helps deliver baby on train.* The Times of India. https://timesofindia.indiatimes.com/city/nagpur/interning-doctor-helps-deliver-baby-on-train/articleshow/58100789.cms

Shuaib, A., Arian, H., & Shuaib, A. (2020). The increasing role of artificial intelligence in health care: Will robots replace doctors in the future? *International Journal of General Medicine, 13,* 891–896. https://doi.org/10.2147/ijgm.s268093

Siwicki, B. (2021, May 17). *Data interoperability, knowledge interoperability and the learning health system.* Healthcare IT News. https://www.healthcareitnews.com/news/data-interoperability-knowledge-interoperability-and-learning-health-system

Smith, R. (2021, July 5). *Time to assume that health research is fraudulent until proven otherwise?* The BMJ. https://blogs.bmj.com/bmj/2021/07/05/time-to-assume-that-health-research-is-fraudulent-until-proved-otherwise/

Søvold, L. E., Naslund, J. A., Kousoulis, A. A., Saxena, S., Qoronfleh, M. W., Grobler, C., & Münter, L. (2021). Prioritizing the Mental Health and Well-Being of Healthcare Workers: An Urgent Global Public Health Priority. *Frontiers in Public Health, 9*(1), 1–12. frontiersin. https://doi.org/10.3389/fpubh.2021.679397

Statista.com. (2016). *Number hospitals Canada by province 2016.* Statista. https://www.statista.com/statistics/440923/total-number-of-hospital-establishments-in-canada-by-province/

Steger, A. (2019, October 3). *3 ways interoperability can improve patient care.* HealthTech. https://healthtechmagazine.net/article/2019/10/3-ways-interoperability-can-improve-patient-care-perfcon

Sunarti, S., Fadzlul Rahman, F., Naufal, M., Risky, M., Febriyanto, K., & Masnina, R. (2021). Artificial intelligence in healthcare: opportunities and risk for future. *Gaceta Sanitaria, 35*(1), S67–S70. https://doi.org/10.1016/j.gaceta.2020.12.019

Tarlo, S. (2023, April 28). *The rise of artificial intelligence, explained.* Vox. https://www.vox.com/2023/4/28/23702644/artificial-intelligence-machine-learning-technology

Telychko, O. (2023, May 12). *What is interoperability in healthcare and why it is necessary.* CodeIT. https://codeit.us/blog/what-is-interoperability-in-healthcare-and-what-are-its-key-benefits

The future of 3D printing? Inside your body. (2019, December 10). Ohio State Insights. https://insights.osu.edu/science/3d-printing-organs

The Impact of Technology in Healthcare. (2019, June 2). AIMS Education. https://aimseducation.edu/blog/the-impact-of-technology-on-healthcare

Thomas, L. (2022, May 24). *Recent Developments in Health Technology.* News Medical. https://www.news-medical.net/health/Recent-Developments-in-Health-Technology.aspx#7

Tiell, S. (2019, November 15). *Create an Ethics Committee to Keep Your AI Initiative in Check.* Harvard Business Review. https://hbr.org/2019/11/create-an-ethics-committee-to-keep-your-ai-initiative-in-check

TRIARE. (2023, July 7). *Millennials want to be able to have their healthcare consult from the same place they order their....* Medium. https://medium.com/@triare/millennials-want-to-be-able-to-have-their-healthcare-consult-from-the-same-place-they-order-their-8f065db7e82

Tweedy, D. (2018). Physicians are people, too. *Health Affairs, 37*(8), 1337–1338. https://doi.org/10.1377/hlthaff.2018.0803

Vegalatos, A., & Sari Vougioukas, J. C. (2004). *Technology's limitation: A drawback in healthcare information systems' acceptance.* Research Gate. https://www.researchgate.net/publication/254123173_TECHNOLOGY'S_LIMITATIONS_A_DRAWBACK_IN_HEALTHCARE_INFORMATION_SYSTEMS'_ACCEPTANCE

Vollers, T. W.-N., & Dennis, A. (2023, March 9). *AI regulation in healthcare: UK and EU approaches.* Lexology. https://www.lexology.com/library/detail.aspx?g=45639f20-f351-4fdd-921f-9b1f38a977e2

What is Artificial Intelligence (AI)? (2023). IBM. https://www.ibm.com/topics/artificial-intelligence

What is health care data management? (2020, August 27). University of Pittsburg. https://online.shrs.pitt.edu/blog/what-is-health-care-data-management/

What is Machine Learning? (2023). IBM. https://www.ibm.com/topics/machine-learning

Yacoubian, C. (2023, January 25). *Interoperability is happening — why Natural Language Processing is such an essential part of it.* Managed Healthcare Executive. https://www.managedhealthcareexecutive.com/view/interoperability-is-happening-why-natural-language-processing-is-such-an-essential-part-of-it

Yaraghi, N. (2023, June 9). *ChatGPT and health care: Implications for interoperability and fairness.* Brookings. https://www.brookings.edu/articles/chatgpt-and-health-care-implications-for-interoperability-and-fairness/